Updates on Sarcopenia - Advances in the Prevention, Diagnosis, and Management

Edited by Élvio Rúbio Gouveia, Andreas Ihle, Marcelo de Maio Nascimento and Bruna R. Gouveia

Published in London, United Kingdom

Updates on Sarcopenia - Advances in the Prevention, Diagnosis, and Management
http://dx.doi.org/10.5772/intechopen.111255
Edited by Élvio Rúbio Gouveia, Andreas Ihle, Marcelo de Maio Nascimento and Bruna R. Gouveia

Contributors
Chanelle Montpetit, Clio Yuen Man Cheng, Jiaming Chen, Katdel Istifanus Dafup, Leticia Andreina Lozada Tobar, Maryse Fortin, Michael H. Weber, Ning Xi, Santiago David Silva Tobar, Vivian W. Q. Lou, Xin Ma

First published in London, United Kingdom, 2026 by IntechOpen
IntechOpen is the global imprint of INTECHOPEN LIMITED, registered in England and Wales, registration number: 11086078, 167-169 Great Portland Street, London, W1W 5PF, United Kingdom

For EU product safety concerns: IN TECH d.o.o., Prolaz Marije Krucifikse Kozulić 3, 51000 Rijeka, Croatia, info@intechopen.com or visit our website at intechopen.com.

British Library Cataloguing-in-Publication Data
A catalogue record for this book is available from the British Library

Updates on Sarcopenia - Advances in the Prevention, Diagnosis, and Management
Edited by Élvio Rúbio Gouveia, Andreas Ihle, Marcelo de Maio Nascimento and Bruna R. Gouveia
p. cm.
Print ISBN 978-0-85466-980-6
Online ISBN 978-0-85466-979-0
eBook (PDF) ISBN 978-0-85466-981-3

Meet the editors

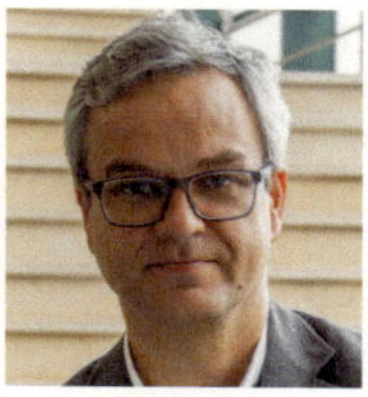

Élvio Rúbio Gouveia is an Associate Professor in the Department of Physical Education and Sport at the University of Madeira and an integrated member of the Interactive Technologies Institute (Robotics and Engineering Systems Laboratory), where he serves as Principal Investigator. He collaborates with the Interdisciplinary Center for the Study of Human Performance at the University of Lisbon. He is an associate member of the Swiss Center of Expertise in Life Course Research (LIVES) and the Center for the Interdisciplinary Study of Gerontology and Vulnerability (CIGEV) at the University of Geneva. He holds a Ph.D. in Sports Sciences from the University of Madeira. His research focuses on healthy aging, sports training, and assistive technologies, with more than 200 articles in peer-reviewed journals.

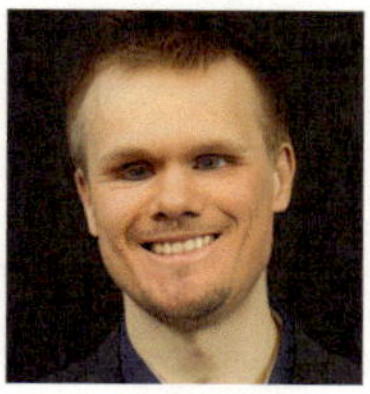

Andreas Ihle is a Professor at the University of Geneva, Switzerland. He received his MSc in Psychology from the University of Dresden, Germany, and his Ph.D. in Psychology from the University of Geneva. His interdisciplinary research focuses on better understanding human development across the lifespan, such as explaining the enormous inter- and intraindividual differences in cognitive functioning, health, well-being, activity engagement, reserve accumulation, and vulnerability from early childhood to late adulthood. On these topics, he has published several articles in international peer-reviewed journals. He is a reviewer for a wide variety of scientific journals and funding agencies.

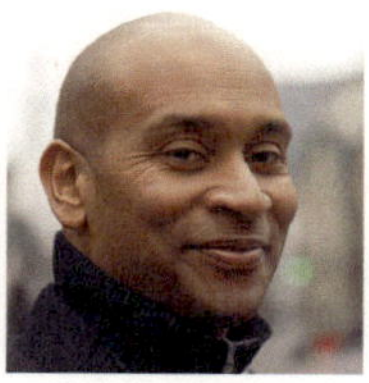

Marcelo de Maio Nascimento holds a Ph.D. in Human Movement Sciences (Cologne University of Physical Education/ Germany). Professor at the Faculty of Physical Education of the Federal University of the São Francisco Valley (UNIVASF), in the Northeast region of Brazil. Researcher in the area of Gerontology of Human Movement, with emphasis on cognition, depression, and frailty. Currently, he is the coordinator of the University of the Third Age (UNATI/UNIVASF).

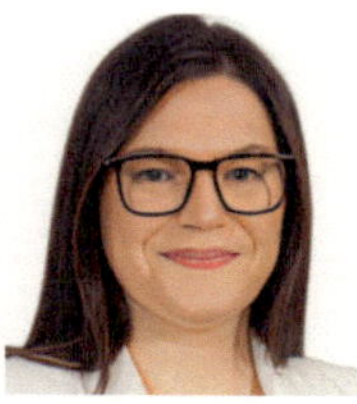

Bruna Raquel Gouveia (BRG) is an Adjunct Professor at the Saint Joseph of Cluny Higher School of Nursing, where she coordinates the Master\'s Program in Rehabilitation Nursing. She is a researcher at ITI – LARSyS and CIGEV at the University of Geneva. She has been the Regional Director of Health in the Autonomous Region of Madeira since 2023, coordinating the design of the region\'s health policies. Her research has focused on human development and aging, as well as the evaluation of complex interventions in rehabilitation and health. Currently, BRG is conducting epidemiological research and developing and implementing innovative health technologies. One example was the use of smart information systems for COVID-19 epidemiological surveillance in Madeira.

Contents

Preface

Sarcopenia, the progressive loss of skeletal muscle mass, strength, and function, has moved from the margins of geriatric research to the center of contemporary medicine. Once dismissed as an inevitable feature of advancing age, it is now recognized as a treatable muscle disease with profound consequences for falls, frailty, surgical outcomes, hospitalization, chronic disease, and mortality. The gap between what is known about sarcopenia and what is consistently done in clinical practice, however, remains too wide. This book was conceived to help close that gap. Rather than aspiring to encyclopedic coverage, it offers a focused, contemporary, and clinically oriented selection of contributions that show where the field stands today and where it is heading. The chapters are organized into three thematic sections: foundational concepts and general approaches to sarcopenia; sarcopenia in distinct clinical contexts, including falls in community-dwelling older adults, degenerative spinal disease, and chronic kidney disease on hemodialysis; and the technological frontier, where wearable sensors, instrumented balance platforms, and machine-learning analytics are extending diagnosis beyond the specialized laboratory.

Three editorial commitments run through the book: fidelity to current international consensus while remaining attentive to its limitations; deliberate inclusion of perspectives and original data from regions and populations; and emphasis on the clinical translation of evidence into assessment, intervention, and the preservation of autonomy for older adults. The intended audience reflects the interdisciplinary nature of the topic: geriatricians, internists, surgeons, nephrologists, rehabilitation specialists, nutritionists, exercise scientists, public-health professionals, postgraduate students, and policy-makers concerned with healthy aging. Sincere thanks are due to the contributing authors, participants, institutions, reviewers, and editorial teams who made the book possible. The aspiration is straightforward: that earlier, smarter, and more equitable approaches to sarcopenia may extend the years of life worth living.

Élvio Rúbio Gouveia
Department of Physical Education and Sport,
University of Madeira,
Madeira, Portugal

Andreas Ihle
University of Geneva,
Geneva, Switzerland

Marcelo de Maio Nascimento
Department of Physical Education,
Federal University of Vale do São Francisco,
Petrolina, Brazil

Bruna R. Gouveia
Nursing School of St. José de Cluny,
Funchal, Portugal

Chapter 1

Quantitative Methods for User-Centered Sarcopenia Identification and Management

Clio Yuen Man Cheng, Vivian W.Q. Lou, Xin Ma, Jiaming Chen and Ning Xi

Abstract

This study aimed to develop a faster and simpler user-centered approach for sarcopenia identification and management using a novel balance sensor system and wearable robots. The study design was a cross-sectional study. The research was conducted based on a community-based study in Hong Kong. A total of 144 community-dwelling older adults were included. Sarcopenia was defined according to the guidelines published by the Asian Working Group for Sarcopenia 2019. Appendicular skeletal muscle mass was calculated using the Lee equation. Among the 46 features extracted from the balance sensor system, 15 displayed a sensitivity >0.8 through a machine-learning approach. The area under the receiver operating characteristics curve of the logistic model in discriminating sarcopenia was 0.68. This study demonstrated that a novel balance sensor system proved useful in sarcopenia identification in older adults. Furthermore, the balance sensor data were valuable in informing the development of wearable robots for sarcopenia management.

Keywords: older adults, physiological, behavioral, functional, quantitative methods, electromyography, balance sensor

1. Introduction

Sarcopenia has been recognized as a disease by the World Health Organization (WHO) under the International Statistical Classification of Diseases and Related Health Problems (ICD), with the code ICD-10-CM (M62.84) [1]. The recognition of sarcopenia as a disease has prompted extensive research endeavors aimed at determining optimal approaches for its screening, diagnosis, and management [2, 3]. Despite concerted efforts, there was no standard definition of sarcopenia until 2024 [4]. According to the latest Delphi consensus from the Global Leadership Initiative in Sarcopenia (GLIS), the conceptual definition of sarcopenia "comprises the concurrent combination of reduced muscle mass and muscle strength" [5]. In a broader sense, sarcopenia is a generalized disease of skeletal muscle with a higher prevalence among older adults. It has been estimated to influence 10–16% of older adults worldwide, particularly in the Asia and Pacific region [6].

Muscle mass depletion in older adults can result in the reduction of up to one-third of their former muscle mass, which is recognized to contribute to gait disorders and, ultimately, incidents of falls [7]. Age-related changes in skeletal muscle composition manifest in a reduced quantity of muscle fibers observed in elderly individuals, particularly notable within the lower limbs, compared to their younger counterparts [8]. Sarcopenia has been considered a significant contributor to musculoskeletal impairments, encompassing disruptions in muscle innervation and neuronal control [9]. Consequently, these factors ultimately impact postural stability, rendering the execution of functional activities that necessitate strength for balance and postural control challenging [10]. A prior meta-analysis revealed that low muscle mass was associated with worsening activities of daily living (ADL) and instrumental activities of daily living (IADL), impacting community-dwelling older adults to maintain independence in late life [11].

Muscle strength reduction imposes a range of negative consequences that significantly impact individuals' lives. As age-related muscle loss occurs, it leads to a decline in physical strength and functional abilities, making daily activities increasingly challenging [11]. Simple tasks such as standing up from a chair, climbing stairs, or carrying objects become more difficult, elevating the risk of falls and injuries [12]. Sarcopenia also contributes to decreased mobility and balance [13], further limiting independence and increasing reliance on assistance from others. Furthermore, the decrease in muscle mass and strength can lead to a reduced metabolic rate [14], increasing the likelihood of weight gain and the risk of chronic conditions like obesity, diabetes, and cardiovascular diseases. Additionally, sarcopenia is associated with an increased susceptibility to frailty [15], decreased bone density [16], and a compromised immune system [17], heightening vulnerability to infections and prolonging recovery times. The psychological impact of sarcopenia should not be overlooked, as it can result in diminished self-esteem [18], heightened dependency [19], and a diminished sense of overall well-being [20].

Traditionally, sarcopenia is assessed using methods such as dual-energy X-ray absorptiometry (DXA) for measuring muscle mass, handgrip strength tests for evaluating muscle strength, and the Short Physical Performance Battery (SPPB) for assessing physical performance [5, 21]. However, these methods have limitations, including a lack of specificity in capturing functional aspects, limited accessibility in different settings, unsuitability for diverse populations, and the inability to capture longitudinal changes [22, 23]. Overcoming these challenges and developing improved assessment techniques is crucial for accurate and comprehensive evaluations of sarcopenia, leading to better management and interventions for those affected. In light of these negative consequences, early identification in community-dwelling older adults is necessary, and novel tools that can be easily applied and operated in daily practice are useful.

Despite the advancements in the definition and recognition of sarcopenia, there remains a significant gap in the literature regarding the development and validation of accessible, cost-effective, and easy-to-use tools for early identification and assessment of sarcopenia in community-dwelling older adults. Existing methods are often resource-intensive, lack functional specificity, and are not suitable for diverse populations or settings. This study aims to address these gaps by proposing a novel assessment tool that is both practical and effective for use in daily practice. Our proposed tool is designed to be easily operable, cost-effective, and capable of capturing functional aspects of sarcopenia that are critical for early diagnosis and intervention. By validating this tool, we hope to provide a reliable method for healthcare providers to identify sarcopenia early in community-dwelling older adults, thereby improving management outcomes and reducing the burden of sarcopenia-related complications.

2. Methods

2.1 Design and participants

This study employed a cross-sectional design. Participants were asked to complete a self-administered survey about their self-reported signs suggestive of sarcopenia, which includes five components: strength, walking, rising from a chair, climbing stairs, and falls. Muscle strength, physical performance, and muscle mass were measured with the assistance of trained research assistants and postgraduate students in university laboratories.

Participants were recruited from the community-dwelling older population in two distinct waves. Initially, between July and August 2021, we enrolled 91 healthy older adults to serve as the reference group. Inclusion criteria for participation included: (1) aged 65 or above, (2) SARC-F score (a measure of sarcopenia potential) below 4, (3) residing in the community in Hong Kong (i.e., not residing in any long-term care facilities), (4) absence of self-reported cognitive impairments, (5) able to engage in a laboratory setting independently, and (6) willing to participate voluntarily. To ensure safety during the experiment, individuals with self-reported osteoporosis and/or a history of spine, knee, hip, or ankle joint surgeries were excluded. Subsequently, between December 2021 and December 2022, we recruited 66 older adults as the user group. Similar inclusion and exclusion criteria were applied to the user group as those stipulated for the reference group, with the exception that 40 of them reported a SARC-F score ≥ 4. Ethical approval was obtained from the Human Research Ethics Committee of the University (EA1903040). All participants were informed that their involvement was entirely voluntary and that they could decline or withdraw at any time. All participants signed an informed consent form.

After a careful data quality check, we removed seven participants from subsequent analyses. Sensitivity analyses were conducted between the removed cases ($n = 7$) and the included cases ($n = 144$), and results indicated no significant differences ($p > .05$) in demographics, muscle strength, physical performance, and muscle between the two groups.

2.2 Diagnostic indicators for sarcopenia

According to the latest guideline of the Asian Working Group for Sarcopenia (AWGS), muscle strength, physical performance, and muscle mass are three important indicators to define sarcopenia. Particularly, "sarcopenia" refers to older adults with low muscle mass and low muscle strength *or* low physical performance; and "severe sarcopenia" refers to older adults with low muscle mass, low muscle strength, *and* low physical performance [21].

Muscle mass, or the appendicular skeletal muscle mass (ASM), was estimated using the Lee equation, following a height-adjustment model [24]: $\text{ASM} = (0.244 \times \text{body weight} + 7.8 \text{ x height} + 6.6 \times \text{gender} - 0.098 \times \text{age} - 4.5)/\text{height}^2$, where gender = 0 for women and one for men. The recommended cutoff for low height-adjusted muscle mass was <7.0 kg/m^2 for men and < 5.7 kg/m^2 for women.

Muscle strength was assessed following the standard procedure using a hand dynamometer [25]. Participants were required to perform three measurements using both hands, and the highest recorded value out of the six measurements was considered. The threshold for determining low muscle strength was set at <28 kg for men and <18 kg for women.

Physical performance was measured using the SPPB [26, 27]. The SPPB evaluates different aspects of physical outcomes in the lower extremities. It includes assessments of static balance in various positions (side-by-side, semi-tandem, and full tandem) for a duration of up to 10 seconds each. Additionally, it measures the ability to perform a 5-time sit-to-stand and determines the gait speed over a 4-meter distance. The scores on the SPPB range from 0 to 12, with higher scores indicating better physical function in the lower extremities. Low physical performance is defined as having a 4-meter gait speed of <1.0 m/s, a time of ≥12 s for completing the five repeated chair stands, or an SPPB score ≤ 9 [21].

2.3 Balance sensor system design

Our team has developed a novel measurement approach utilizing a balance sensor system based on the FTIR principle [28]. This system, depicted in **Figure 1**, has been designed to accurately measure the pressure distribution beneath an individual's feet. The system comprises two transparent glass optic-wave guides and a high-resolution wireless camera. By directing LED light into the edges of the glass plates, the disrupted internal reflection upon foot contact enables the camera to capture diffused light at the points of contact. These images are then wirelessly transmitted to a computer, enabling real-time visualization of the pressure distribution. The sensor's innovative design incorporates glass plates set at a 45-degree angle, incorporating mirrors to reflect images to the camera. This design not only enhances image clarity but also ensures a more compact and user-safe device.

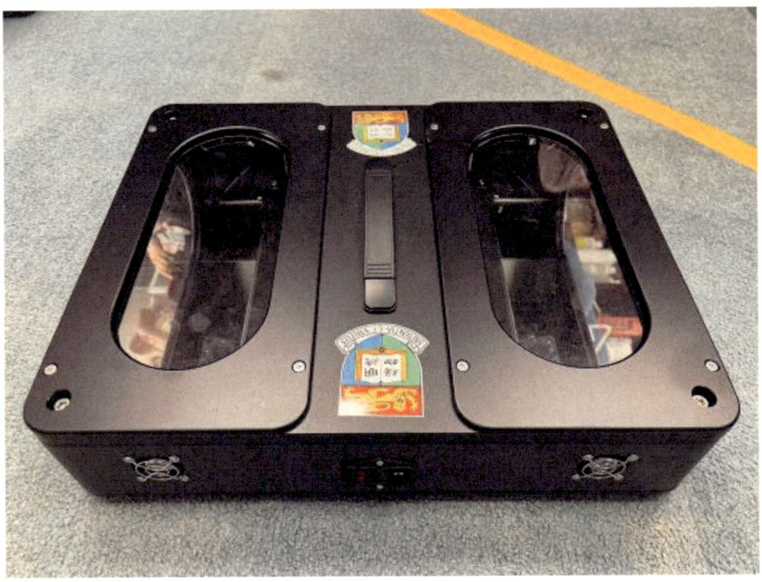

Figure 1.
Balance sensor design.

When pressure is exerted on the surface of inhomogeneous and microscopically deformable latex rubber, its conformity to the contacting glass surface is enhanced, resulting in an increased contact area. Consequently, this enlargement leads to a linear rise in the density of near-contact spots, as demonstrated in **Figure 2**. In the setup employing the FTIR technique, the intensity of diffused light directly corresponds to the microscopic contact area between the latex and the glass. This intensity is captured as pixel values by a charged-coupled device (CCD) camera, where the diffused light intensity is proportionately reflected.

To quantitatively describe the relationship between the intensity of diffused light (I) and the applied pressure (P), a power function model is chosen. The fitting of this model to the collected data is illustrated in **Figure 3**. By calculating the differences (residuals) between the observed values and the model's predictions and optimizing the parameters a and b to minimize the sum of squares of these residuals, the optimal

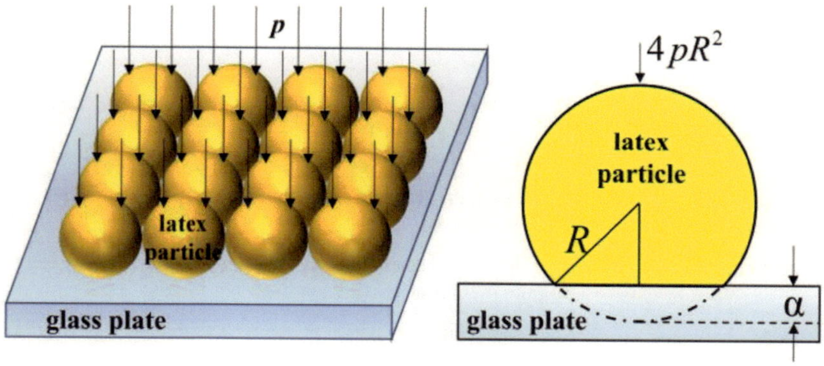

Figure 2.
Ball contact model of later rubber and glass plate.

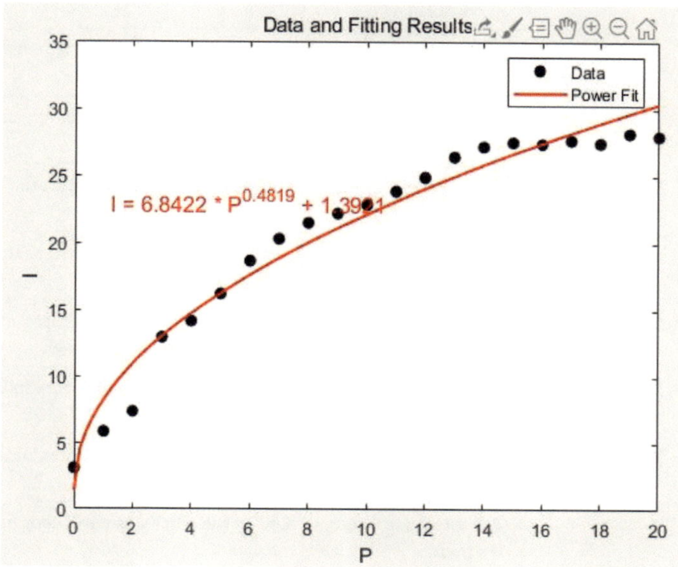

Figure 3.
The relationship between I and P using a power function.

model parameters can be determined. This approach, known as the "Least Squares" principle, is employed to identify the model parameters that best describe the observed relationship. The left graph in the diagram represents the theoretical model, while the right graph presents the results obtained from this modeling approach.

2.4 Experiment procedure and balance sensor features

During the experiment, participants were instructed to remove their shoes and socks and stand barefoot on the designated plates, allowing the balance sensor to detect even subtle changes in balance and pressure distribution. They were asked to maintain a still stance, gaze straight ahead, and keep their hands alongside their bodies for 30 seconds. This specific posture ensured accurate recording of shifts in the center of pressure, providing valuable insights into participants' balance and stability. The collected data played a crucial role in evaluating the effectiveness and sensitivity of the balance sensor.

Variables	Descriptions
ellipse_area_ gravity_center_X_ gravity_center_Y	The area of the confidence ellipse for the gravity center coordinates (X, Y).
range_of_excursion_ gravity_center_X	The range of the gravity center X coordinates, indicating the maximum horizontal movement.
gravity_center_X_ rms	The root mean square of the gravity center X coordinate, a measure of the magnitude of variations.
gravity_center_X_ sample_entropy	The sample entropy of the gravity center X coordinate indicates the complexity or unpredictability of the X coordinate.
gravity_center_X_ band_power	The band power of the gravity center X coordinates, reflecting the power within a specific frequency band.
path_length	The total path length of the movement represents the distance traveled by the gravity center.
velocity	The average velocity is calculated as the total path length divided by the total time of the movement.
acceleration	The average acceleration is calculated as the change in velocity over the time interval.
gravity_center_X _mean	The mean of the gravity center X coordinate, represents the average horizontal position.
gravity_center_X _median	The median of the gravity center X coordinate, represents the middle value in the distribution of X coordinates.
gravity_center_X _std	The standard deviation of the gravity center X coordinate, measuring the variability or dispersion around the mean X coordinate.
gravity_center_X _max	The maximum value of the gravity center X coordinates, indicating the furthest right position reached.
gravity_center_X _min	The minimum value of the gravity center X coordinates, indicating the furthest left position reached.
gravity_center_X _iqr	The interquartile range (IQR) of the gravity center X coordinate, measuring the middle 50% range of the data.

Table 1.
Selected features related to the center of pressure (CoP) and center of gravity (CoG).

For safety purposes, handles were provided on both sides of the setup to assist participants in maintaining balance and offering support if they felt unsteady during the test. Trained research assistants closely monitored the procedure, ready to intervene and provide assistance if any participant experienced discomfort or instability. The center of pressure (CoP), represented by coordinates on the X and Y axes, was analyzed using the digitized output signals from the balance sensor. The time series data captured the path of the CoP relative to the origin of the sensor, with the final 30 seconds of the test period (900 points) used to compute measures in both the time and frequency domains. By combining the balance sensor with a biomechanical model, a comprehensive set of 46 features related to the CoP and the center of gravity (CoG) was extracted across both domains, as detailed in **Table 1**.

Support Vector Machines (SVM) represent a robust classification method that exhibits resilience when dealing with instances where data points are initially nonlinearly separable [29, 30]. By leveraging the kernel trick, SVM facilitates the projection of input data into a feature space of higher dimensionality, thereby simplifying the separation of data points. Within this transformed space, the algorithm identifies a hyperplane that optimizes the margin between the closest points from distinct classes, referred to as support vectors. These vectors play a pivotal role as they establish the boundaries of the decision surface. Once the optimal hyperplane is determined, it is then mapped back to the original space to classify new data points. SVM demonstrates notable efficacy in high-dimensional scenarios characterized by distinct class separability. However, challenges arise when confronted with extensive datasets or situations in which class boundaries overlap, attributable to the computational demands and the complexities involved in identifying an effective separation margin.

3. Results

3.1 Participant characteristics

The data for this study were collected from a sample of 144 older adults residing in the community, with ages ranging from 65 to 84 years (M = 69.44 years, SD = 3.78). Approximately two-thirds of the participants were female (n = 92) and married (n = 92). Among these 144 older adults, 23 (16.0%) were classified as sarcopenia according to the AWGS guideline [21]. **Table 2** summarizes the demographic characteristics.

	Non-sarcopenia (n =121)	Sarcopenia (n = 23)	Statistics
Age (M, SD)	69.56 (3.82)	68.78 (3.55)	$t(142) = .91$
Gender***			X^2 (1) = 15.47
Female	69 (57.0%)	23 (100.0%)	
Male	52 (43.0%)	0 (0.0%)	
Marital status			X^2 (1) = 5.07
Never married	10 (8.3%)	4 (17.4%)	
Married	76 (62.8%)	16 (69.6%)	

	Non-sarcopenia (n =121)	Sarcopenia (n = 23)	Statistics
Widowed	18 (14.9%)	3 (13.0%)	
Separated	5 (4.1%)	0 (0.0%)	
Divorced	12 (9.9%)	0 (0.0%)	
Education			X^2 (4) = 3.29
Primary or below	22 (18.2%)	5 (21.7%)	
Secondary	57 (47.1%)	14 (60.9%)	
Postsecondary	22 (18.2%)	2 (8.7%)	
Undergraduate	12 (9.9%)	1 (4.3%)	
Postgraduate	8 (6.6%)	1 (4.3%)	
Financial situation			X^2 (3) = 2.34
Very insufficient	4 (3.3%)	0 (0.0%)	
Insufficient	27 (22.4%)	4 (17.4%)	
Sufficient	85 (70.2%)	19 (82.6%)	
Very sufficient	5 (4.1%)	0 (0.0%)	
Experienced fall(s)	38 (31.4%)	6 (26.1%)	X^2 (1) = .548

Note: $^{*}p < .05$, $^{**}p < .01$, $^{***}p < .001$.

Table 2.
Participant characteristics by sarcopenia status (N = 144).

3.2 Diagnostic characteristics

The descriptive results of diagnostic characteristics according to the AWGS [21] are presented in **Table 3**.

3.3 Balance sensor features validation

After completing the experiment using the balance sensor system, the prevalence of sarcopenia within the participant group was determined. Our analysis focused specifically on the sensitivity of various features concerning sarcopenia classification. Notably, 15 features displayed a sensitivity exceeding 0.8, as depicted in **Figures 4** and **5**.

To provide a visual representation of these findings, we constructed box plots and ROC curves that illustrate the discriminative power of sensor features in sarcopenia classifications, consistent with AWGS guidelines [21] (see **Figure 6**).

Furthermore, our study employed the SVM algorithm to analyze and identify selected features of the elderly, utilizing short 10-second and 30-second videos from a dataset comprising 144 older adults. The SVM algorithm was specifically tailored to maximize classification accuracy with a focus on fall history, a critical risk factor in geriatric care. Notably, under a random state of 56, the SVM model exhibited a sensitivity of 82.9% in correctly identifying individuals with a fall history. This sensitivity improved to 87% under a random state of 78, highlighting the model's strong capability in detecting true positive cases, which is essential for

DOI: http://dx.doi.org/10.5772/intechopen.1005848

	Non-sarcopenia (n = 121)	Sarcopenia (n = 23)	Statistics
Muscle mass			
Skeletal muscle mass (kg/m^2), (M, SD)***	7.52 (1.49)	4.98 (.35)	$t(142) = 8.110$
High: m: ≥7 kg/m^2; f: ≥5.7 kg/m^2	117 (96.7%)	0 (0.0%)	X^2 (1) = 118.612
Low: m: <7 kg/m^2; f: <5.7 kg/m^2	4 (3.3%)	23 (100.0%)	
Muscle strength			
Maximum handgrip strength (kg), (M, SD)***	25.23 (8.81)	17.79 (4.95)	$t(142) = 3.929$
High: m: ≥28 kg; f: ≥18 kg	82 (67.8%)	11 (47.8%)	X^2 (1) = 3.360
Low: m: <28 kg; f: <18 kg	39 (32.2%)	12 (52.2%)	
Physical performance			
SPPB total score (0–12)	10.59 (1.82)	10.09 (2.02)	$t(142) = 1.184$
High: >9	91 (75.2%)	15 (65.2%)	X^2 (1) = .993
Low: ≤9	30 (24.8%)	8 (34.8%)	
Average 4-m gait speed (m/s), (M, SD)	.83 (.26)	.73 (.21)	$t(142) = 1.676$
High: ≥1.0 m/s**	33 (27.3%)	1 (4.3%)	X^2 (1) = 5.631
Low: <1.0 m/s	88 (72.7%)	22 (95.7%)	
Average time for 5-time sit-to-stand (s)	10.95 (5.08)	11.97 (3.88)	$t(140) = -.913$
High: <12 s*	79 (65.3%)	10 (43.5%)	X^2 (1) = 3.895
Low: ≥12 s	42 (34.7%)	13 (56.5%)	
Physical performance@***			X^2 (1) = 5.631
High	33 (27.3%)	1 (4.3%)	
Low	88 (72.7%)	22 (95.7%)	

Note. *$p < .05$.
**$p < .01$.
***$p < .001$.
@*Low physical performance is defined as a 4-m walk speed <1.0 m/s, or a Short Physical Performance Battery (SPPB) score ≤9, or a 5-time sit-to-stand completion time ≥12 s.*

Table 3.
Behavioral level quantitative assessments by sarcopenia status (N = 144).

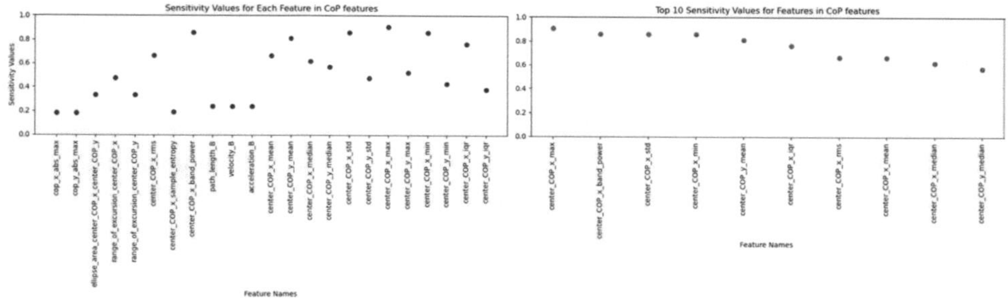

Figure 4.
Sensitivity of the selected features related to the center of pressure (CoP).

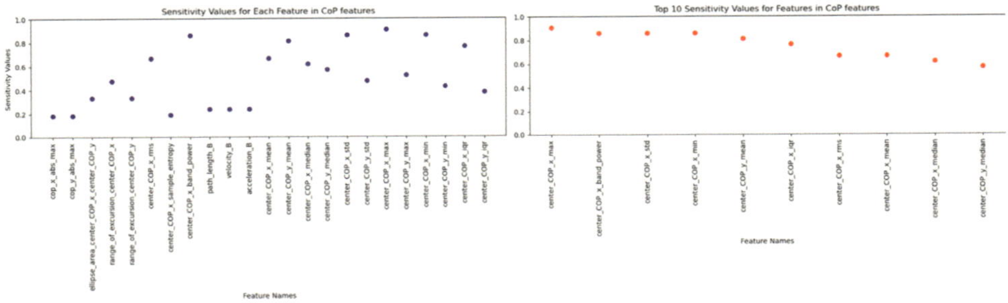

Figure 5.
Sensitivity of the selected features related to the center of gravity (CoG).

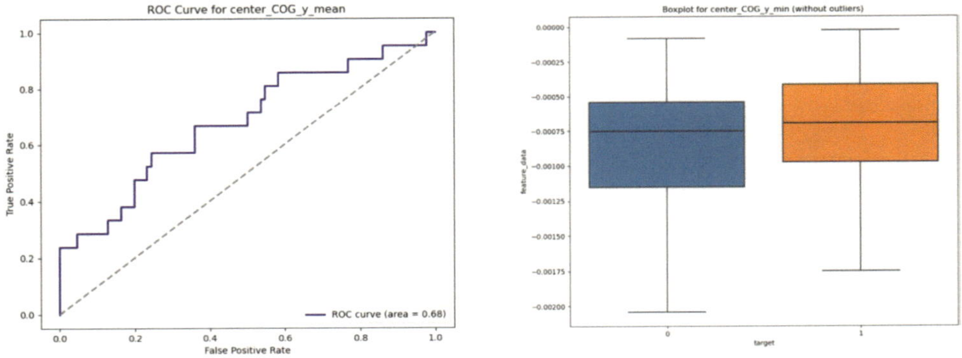

Figure 6.
Box plots and ROC curves that delineate the sensor features' discriminative power over sarcopenia classifications.

effective fall risk assessment. Conversely, the specificity, indicating the model's accuracy in identifying individuals without a fall history, was recorded at 97.5% under a random state of 36 but decreased to 85.3% under a random state of 34. This variation in specificity underscores the model's sensitivity to changes in testing conditions and underscores the importance of meticulous model tuning and validation. The robust performance of the SVM across diverse testing scenarios demonstrates its potential utility in geriatric care, particularly in the realm of fall prevention strategies. The high sensitivity and specificity achieved under different conditions provide a solid foundation for further research and the development of advanced predictive tools in this domain.

4. Discussion

The present study aimed to investigate the potential utility of a novel balance sensor system in user-centered sarcopenia identification. By analyzing various diagnostic characteristics and participant characteristics, valuable insights were obtained regarding the identification and management of sarcopenia in older adults. The findings from the study suggest that the balance sensor system can serve as a useful, faster, and simpler approach for identifying sarcopenia in community-dwelling older adults. The sensitivity analysis of selected features related to the CoP and CoG demonstrated promising results, with 15 features exhibiting high sensitivity, indicating their potential for accurate sarcopenia classification.

DOI: http://dx.doi.org/10.5772/intechopen.1005848

These results have significant implications for user-centered sarcopenia management, particularly in the context of wearable robot development. Wearable robots have shown promise in assisting older adults with mobility and strength-related tasks. By leveraging the data obtained from the balance sensor system, wearable robots can be developed to provide personalized and targeted interventions for individuals with sarcopenia [31–33]. While the balance sensor system cannot directly monitor muscle mass, strength, and physical performance measures in real-time, the extracted features provide valuable information regarding balance and postural control. These features can be indicators of underlying muscle weakness and functional decline associated with sarcopenia.

In the context of wearable robot development, the data obtained from the balance sensor system can contribute to personalized interventions targeting specific aspects of balance and postural control. By leveraging the identified features, wearable robots can be designed to provide targeted exercises and assistance aimed at improving balance, stability, and overall physical function. It is important to note that the balance sensor system is still in its development stage and should be used in conjunction with other assessment methods to comprehensively evaluate sarcopenia. Direct measurements of muscle mass and strength, such as SPPB and handgrip dynamometry, remain essential for accurate diagnosis and monitoring of sarcopenia progression.

The practical implications of these findings are substantial for the management of sarcopenia. The balance sensor system offers a noninvasive, quick, and user-friendly tool that can be used in various settings, including clinics and community centers, to screen for sarcopenia in the general public. Healthcare professionals can incorporate this tool into routine assessments to identify individuals at risk of sarcopenia early and tailor interventions accordingly. Given its simplicity and speed, the balance sensor system can facilitate more frequent monitoring, thereby enabling timely adjustments to treatment plans. Furthermore, older adults could use the balance sensor system for daily monitoring, thus, reducing fall risks and balance-related injuries. Ultimately, to enhance quality of life and reduce medical costs.

Future research should focus on further validating the balance sensor system in larger and more diverse populations to ensure its generalizability. Additionally, integrating balance sensor data with other direct measurements of muscle mass and strength could provide a more comprehensive assessment of sarcopenia. Research should also explore the development of algorithms that can combine data from multiple sources to improve the accuracy of sarcopenia diagnosis and monitoring.

The study has several limitations. Firstly, the sample size was relatively small and may not be representative of the broader population of older adults. Secondly, the balance sensor system, while showing promise, is still in the development stage and requires further refinement and validation. Thirdly, the study did not include direct comparisons with established diagnostic tools for sarcopenia such as DXA, which could provide a more comprehensive validation of the balance sensor system's effectiveness. Lastly, the system cannot currently monitor muscle mass and strength in real-time, which limits its standalone diagnostic capability.

In summary, while the balance sensor system may not directly monitor muscle mass, strength, and physical performance measures in real-time, it provides valuable information related to balance and postural control. When combined with other assessment methods, the system can contribute to user-centered sarcopenia management and inform the development of wearable robots to enhance balance, stability, and overall physical function. Further research is necessary to explore the integration of balance sensor data with other measurements for a comprehensive approach to sarcopenia assessment and intervention.

5. Conclusions

This study sheds light on the potential of a balance sensor system as a valuable tool for user-centered sarcopenia identification and management. The findings highlight the importance of analyzing diagnostic characteristics and participant characteristics in assessing sarcopenia and guiding interventions. While the balance sensor system provides specific features related to balance and postural control, it can contribute to the development of personalized interventions through wearable robot technology. Future research should focus on integrating the balance sensor data with other assessment methods, such as direct measurements of muscle mass and strength, to provide a more comprehensive evaluation of sarcopenia. Additionally, further exploration is needed to optimize the use of machine-learning algorithms for accurate sarcopenia classification and fall risk assessment. By advancing these areas, we can enhance geriatric care, promote healthy aging, and develop effective strategies for managing sarcopenia in older adults.

Acknowledgements

The authors would like to thank all study participants and the teams at The University of Hong Kong and the City University of Hong Kong. The authors would like to thank all the researchers, students, and research assistants who contributed to the design and execution of the experiments. We would also like to thank all the participants for their time, effort, and valuable feedback. The work described in this paper was fully supported by a grant from the Research Grants Council of the Hong Kong Special Administrative Region, China (Project No. [T42-717/20-R]) and a grant from the Innovation and Technology Commission of the Hong Kong Special Administrative Region, China (Project No. [ITB/FBL/4018/21/P]).

Conflict of interest

The authors declare no conflict of interest.

Author details

Clio Yuen Man Cheng[1,2], Vivian W.Q. Lou[1,2*], Xin Ma[3,4], Jiaming Chen[3,4] and Ning Xi[3,4]

1 Department of Social Work and Social Administration, The University of Hong Kong, Hong Kong, China

2 Sau Po Centre on Ageing, The University of Hong Kong, Hong Kong, China

3 Department of Industrial and Manufacturing Systems Engineering, The University of Hong Kong, Hong Kong, China

4 Advanced Technologies Institute, The University of Hong Kong, Hong Kong, China

*Address all correspondence to: wlou@hku.hk

References

[1] Anker SD, Morley JE, von Haehling S. Welcome to the ICD-10 code for sarcopenia. Journal of Cachexia, Sarcopenia and Muscle. 2016;7(5):512-514. DOI: 10.1002/jcsm.12147

[2] Beaudart C, Zaaria M, Pasleau F, Reginster J-Y, Bruyère O. Health outcomes of sarcopenia: A systematic review and meta-analysis. PLoS One. 2017;**12**(1):e0169548. DOI: 10.1371/journal.pone.0169548

[3] Xie W-Q, Xiao G-L, Hu P-W, He Y-Q, Lv S, Xiao W-F. Possible sarcopenia: Early screening and intervention-narrative review. Annals of Palliative Medicine. 2020:46-46. DOI: 10.21037/apm-20-967

[4] Alhmly HF, Fielding RA. A critical review of current worldwide definitions of sarcopenia. Calcified Tissue International. Jan 2024;**114**(1):74-81. DOI: 10.1007/s00223-023-01163-3. Epub 2023 Dec 3. PMID: 38043100

[5] Kirk B et al. The conceptual definition of sarcopenia: Delphi consensus from the global leadership initiative in sarcopenia (GLIS). Age and Ageing. 2024;**53**(3):afae052. DOI: 10.1093/ageing/afae052

[6] Yuan S, Larsson SC. Epidemiology of sarcopenia: Prevalence, risk factors, and consequences. Metabolism. 2023;**144**:155533. DOI: 10.1016/j.metabol.2023.155533

[7] Jørstad EC, Hauer K, Becker C, Lamb SE, on behalf of the P. Group. Measuring the psychological outcomes of falling: A systematic review. Journal of the American Geriatrics Society. 2005;**53**(3):501-510. DOI: 10.1111/j.1532-5415.2005.53172.x

[8] Venturelli M et al. In vivo and in vitro evidence that intrinsic upper- and lower-limb skeletal muscle function is unaffected by ageing and disuse in oldest-old humans. Acta Physiologica. 2015;**215**(1):58-71. DOI: 10.1111/apha.12524

[9] Cruz-Jentoft AJ, Sayer AA. Sarcopenia. Lancet. 2019;**393**(10191):2636-2646. DOI: 10.1016/s0140-6736(19)31138-9

[10] Kim AY, Lee JK, Kim SH, Choi J, Song JJ, Chae SW. Is postural dysfunction related to sarcopenia? A population-based study. PLoS One. 2020;**15**(5):e0232135. DOI: 10.1371/journal.pone.0232135

[11] Wang DXM, Yao J, Zirek Y, Reijnierse EM, Maier AB. Muscle mass, strength, and physical performance predicting activities of daily living: A meta-analysis. Journal of Cachexia, Sarcopenia and Muscle. 2019;**11**(1):3-25. DOI: 10.1002/jcsm.12502

[12] Rodrigues F, Domingos C, Monteiro D, Morouço P. A review on aging, sarcopenia, falls, and resistance training in community-dwelling older adults. International Journal of Environmental Research and Public Health. 2022;**19**(2):874. DOI: 10.3390/ijerph19020874

[13] Kato T, Ikezoe T, Tabara Y, Matsuda F, Tsuboyama T, Ichihashi N. Differences in lower limb muscle strength and balance ability between sarcopenia stages depend on sex in community-dwelling older adults. Aging Clinical and Experimental Research. 2022;**34**(3):527-534. DOI: 10.1007/s40520-021-01952-6

[14] Soysal P, Ates Bulut E, Yavuz I, Isik AT. Decreased basal metabolic rate

can be an objective marker for sarcopenia and frailty in older males. Journal of the American Medical Directors Association. 2019;**20**(1):58-63. DOI: 10.1016/j.jamda.2018.07.001

[15] Chau A, Kim DH, Sison SDM, Shi SM. Mobility device use and frailty progression in community-dwelling older adults with mobility limitations. Journal of Aging and Health. 2 Apr 2024:08982643241242927. DOI: 10.1177/08982643241242927. PMID: 38565230 [Epub ahead of print]

[16] Cheng L, Wang S. Correlation between bone mineral density and sarcopenia in US adults: A population-based study. Journal of Orthopaedic Surgery. 2023;**18**(1):588. DOI: 10.1186/s13018-023-04034-7

[17] Zhang X, Li H, He M, Wang J, Wu Y, Li Y. Immune system and sarcopenia: Presented relationship and future perspective. Experimental Gerontology. 2022;**164**:111823. DOI: 10.1016/j.exger.2022.111823

[18] Nho J-H, Kim EJ. Factors affecting the quality of life in low-income older adults with sarcopenia: A cross-sectional study. Journal of Korean Academy of Nursing. 2023;**53**(1):1-11. DOI: 10.4040/jkan.22126

[19] Perez-Sousa MA et al. Gait speed as a mediator of the effect of sarcopenia on dependency in activities of daily living. Journal of Cachexia, Sarcopenia and Muscle. 2019;**10**(5):1009-1015. DOI: 10.1002/jcsm.12444

[20] Veronese N et al. Sarcopenia reduces quality of life in the long-term: Longitudinal analyses from the English longitudinal study of ageing. European Geriatric Medicine. 2022;**13**(3):633-639. DOI: 10.1007/s41999-022-00627-3

[21] Chen L-K et al. Asian working group for sarcopenia: 2019 consensus update on sarcopenia diagnosis and treatment. Journal of the American Medical Directors Association. 2020;**21**(3):300-307.e2. DOI: 10.1016/j.jamda.2019.12.012

[22] Cao M et al. Prevalence of sarcopenia under different diagnostic criteria and the changes in muscle mass, muscle strength, and physical function with age in Chinese old adults. BMC Geriatrics. 2022;**22**(1):889. DOI: 10.1186/s12877-022-03601-7

[23] Evans WJ, Guralnik J, Cawthon P, Appleby J, Landi F, Clarke L, et al. Sarcopenia: No consensus, no diagnostic criteria, and no approved indication—How did we get here? Geroscience. Feb 2024;**46**(1):183-190. DOI: 10.1007/s11357-023-01016-9. Epub 2023 Nov 24. PMID: 37996722; PMCID: PMC10828356

[24] Lee RC, Wang Z, Heo M, Ross R, Janssen I, Heymsfield SB. Total-body skeletal muscle mass: Development and cross-validation of anthropometric prediction models. The American Journal of Clinical Nutrition. 2000;**72**(3):796-803. DOI: 10.1093/ajcn/72.3.796

[25] Roberts HC et al. A review of the measurement of grip strength in clinical and epidemiological studies: Towards a standardised approach. Age and Ageing. 2011;**40**(4):423-429. DOI: 10.1093/ageing/afr051

[26] Guralnik JM et al. A short physical performance battery assessing lower extremity function: Association with self-reported disability and prediction of mortality and nursing home admission. Journal of Gerontology. 1994;**49**(2):M85-M94. DOI: 10.1093/geronj/49.2.M85

[27] Guralnik JM et al. Lower extremity function and subsequent disability: Consistency across studies, predictive models, and value of

gait speed alone compared with the short physical performance battery. Journals of Gerontology Series A. 2000;**55**(4):M221-M231. DOI: 10.1093/gerona/55.4.m221

[28] Wang S, Xi N. Recurrent transfer learning by neural network regression for human balance sensor calibration. In: 2019 IEEE Sensors. Montreal, QC, Canada; 2019. pp. 1-4. DOI: 10.1109/SENSORS43011.2019.8956907

[29] Ahsan H, Khandoker DTH, Lai RK, Begg, Palaniswami M. Wavelet-based feature extraction for support vector machines for screening balance impairments in the elderly. IEEE Transactions on Neural Systems and Rehabilitation Engineering. 2007;**15**(4):587-597. DOI: 10.1109/TNSRE.2007.906961

[30] Joshi AV. Support vector machines. In: Joshi AV, editor. Machine Learning and Artificial Intelligence. Cham: Springer International Publishing; 2023. pp. 89-99. DOI: 10.1007/978-3-031-12282-8_8

[31] Lou VWQ, Cheng CYM, Chen K, Or CKL, Hu Y, Xi N. Applying an innovative user-centric co-creation (UC3) approach in developing intelligent wearable robots for elderly assistance: From a transdisciplinary lens. In: Structural Health Monitoring 2023. United States of America: DEStech Publi cations, Inc.; 2023. pp. 2023-2035. [Online]. Available from: https://www.drive.google.com/file/d/1pwr0kOjmj7N-Cp6EBjOomkQIJ-OCXpuQ/view?usp=sharing

[32] Lou VWQ, Cheng CYM, Xi N. Advancing the development of intelligent wearable robots for elderly assistance: An innovative user-centric Co-creation (UC3) framework. In: Presented at the 15th International Conference on Applied Human Factors and Ergonomics, Université Côte d'Azur. Nice, France: AHFE; 2024

[33] Xi N et al. Intelligent Robotics for Elderly Assistance in Hong Kong [Online]. Available from: https://www.ugc.edu.hk/eng/rgc/funding_opport/trs/funded_research/trs10_lay_sum.html#402_20

Chapter 2

The Multifaceted Impact of Skeletal Muscle Morphology and Function on Spine Pathologies

Chanelle Montpetit, Michael H. Weber and Maryse Fortin

Abstract

Skeletal muscle morphometry, quality, and function serve as crucial prognostic indicators across various medical and surgical fields. Sarcopenia, the progressive loss of muscle mass and function, significantly contributes to frailty in individuals with spine pathologies. Abnormalities in spinal muscle mass and function (e.g., sarcopenia) are not only associated with the development of spine-related disorders but also negatively affect quality of life and postoperative outcomes. Tailored treatments and effective pre and post-operative rehabilitation strategies are imperative to mitigate complications, enhance quality of life, and expected survival in patients with diverse spinal pathologies. The intricate relationship between spine pathologies, sarcopenia, and factors like patient-reported health-related quality of life, frailty, surgery-related adverse events, and cost-effectiveness necessitates a comprehensive approach from spine care providers. Recognizing the broader implications of muscle loss on physical function, pain levels, and quality of life is essential for spine care providers to optimize both non-operative and operative care.

Keywords: spine pathologies, musculoskeletal health, skeletal muscle quality, patient-reported health-related quality of life, muscle function, sarcopenia

1. Introduction

1.1 Sarcopenia epidemiology

Sarcopenia, a term derived from the Greek language meaning "loss of flesh," is a silent yet challenging adversary in the field of public health [1]. Coined by Irwin Rosenberg in the 1980s, sarcopenia was defined as the age-related reduction in muscle tissue that can lead to a decline in functional capacity [1]. The European Working Group on Sarcopenia further refined the definition in 2019, describing sarcopenia as a "progressive and generalized skeletal muscle disorder that is associated with increased likelihood of adverse outcomes including falls, fractures, physical disability and mortality" [2]. However, there is a lack of a universally established definition which poses challenges in the assessment of sarcopenia, especially in the context of spinal pathologies. Although aging naturally leads to a decline in skeletal muscle mass and strength, the severity and rate of this loss vary significantly between individuals [3]. Sarcopenia goes beyond this age-related phenomenon, encompassing various factors contributing to its etiology [3].

The prevalence of sarcopenia differs across populations and demographic groups, providing a complex perspective of the disease's global impact, including its implications for spinal health [3, 4]. Studies consistently highlight a higher prevalence among the elderly, with estimates suggesting that a significant proportion of individuals over the age of 60 experience some degree of muscle degradation, potentially impacting the musculature that supports the spine [3]. In communities with older, more complex, or severely ill individuals, the incidence of sarcopenia was found to be higher, introducing additional considerations for spinal health in these populations [4, 5]. The development of sarcopenia is influenced by a myriad of factors that extend beyond the ticking hands of time. Genetic disposition, physical activity levels, nutritional factors, and chronic medical conditions are among the multifaceted risk factors contributing to the onset or worsening of the condition [3]. Age-related changes in muscle fibers, motor units, and neuromuscular junctions, which are integral to spinal stability, predispose individuals to develop sarcopenia [3]. Hormones such as estrogen, testosterone, growth hormone (GH), and insulin-like growth factor-1 (IGF-1) play a vital role in maintaining muscle mass and function, suggesting that disruptions in these hormones can not only contribute to sarcopenia, but also impact the health of muscles supporting the spine [3, 4]. Additionally, malnutrition, insufficient protein intake, age-related changes in appetite and metabolism, sedentary lifestyles, and physical inactivity are all linked to decreased muscle mass and an increased risk of sarcopenia [3]. Lastly, certain medical conditions can contribute to sarcopenia by inducing inflammatory processes, limiting physical activity, and altering muscle metabolism [3, 4]. Sarcopenia is a multidimensional condition driven by complex changes, ultimately impacting the health of the spine [3].

Beyond its physiological toll, sarcopenia imposes a substantial economic burden on healthcare systems worldwide, and its implications extend to the realm of spinal health. The costs associated with the diagnosis, treatment, and management of sarcopenia are compounded by the secondary consequences of related health issues, such as falls, fractures, and hospitalizations [3]. According to estimates, a 10% decrease in the prevalence of sarcopenia could result in an annual reduction of 1.1 billion dollars in healthcare costs in the United States alone [5]. As the global population ages and the incidence of spine pathologies rises simultaneously, an impending economic burden is poised to escalate, necessitating proactive solutions.

The challenge of addressing the economic burden is compounded by the lack of a universally accepted definition, leading to variations in assessment criteria [6]. Various methods are used to evaluate sarcopenia, specifically relevant in the context of spine pathologies. Imaging techniques such as magnetic resonance imaging (MRI) scans, computerized tomography (CT) scans, dual-energy-X-ray absorptiometry scans, and bioelectrical impedance analysis, assess skeletal muscle mass by measuring cross-sectional area or volume [3, 5]. Muscle strength is assessed through handgrip strength and isokinetic strength testing [3, 5]. Functional performance tests (e.g., Timed Up and Go, Chair Stand Test) evaluate overall physical function [3, 5]. Serum biomarkers (i.e., creatinine and myostatin) serve as indicators of muscle health [7]. Lastly, composite indices, known as sarcopenia indices, combine measures of muscle mass, strength, and physical performance for a comprehensive evaluation [8]. Despite the common use of these methods, the lack of a universally accepted definition has led to variability in assessment criteria, with considerations for population differences (e.g., older adults, individuals with spine pathologies). Researchers and clinicians must navigate these nuances and select appropriate measures based on the context, while ongoing efforts aim to establish standardized criteria for sarcopenia assessments.

1.2 Skeletal muscle health in healthcare

Skeletal muscle, often relegated to a supporting role in health, is emerging as a fundamental component of medicine and surgery, carrying significant implications for patient outcomes and treatment efficacy [9]. Accounting for approximately 40% of the human body, skeletal muscle extends far beyond its obvious function as a locomotor system [10]. Its significance permeates all aspects of health, influencing metabolism, immune function, and overall physiological well-being [10]. The role of skeletal muscle gains particular importance as it plays a crucial role in supporting the spine's structure and function [9, 11, 12]. The muscles surrounding the spine, including the paraspinal muscles, contribute to spinal stability and proper alignment [9, 13].

Medical and surgical outcomes hinge on skeletal muscle health, as it impacts patient resilience, recovery, and long-term prognosis [14]. Skeletal muscle health serves as a barometer of systematic well-being and spinal health. Research indicates that compromised skeletal muscle health is often associated with spinal conditions, reducing the effectiveness of treatments and surgical outcomes [15]. Reduced muscle mass and function around the spine are indicative of underlying issues, ranging from chronic spinal diseases to nutritional deficiencies [13, 14]. Consequently, physicians specializing in spinal care should leverage skeletal muscle assessments to gauge the disease severity, monitor progression, and develop tailored treatment plans that address the spine and its supporting musculature [9].

Beyond diagnostics, healthy spine muscles play a preventive role in various health complications, contributing to quality of life [13]. Surgical interventions, ranging from routine procedures to complex spinal surgeries rely on skeletal muscle health [14]. Preoperative muscle assessments are crucial for physicians to evaluate surgical risk, particularly in patients with pre-existing conditions. Skeletal muscle health is also vital for postoperative recovery, wound healing, and surgical success [16]. During the postoperative phase, the health of spine skeletal muscles influence the speed and efficacy of rehabilitation, shaping the overall trajectory of recovery.

Spine muscle health profoundly impacts functional outcomes in both medical and surgical contexts. Spine muscular strength and endurance are integral components of daily activities and independent living [13, 14]. Postoperative rehabilitation heavily relies on restoring spine and core muscle function, emphasizing the connection between musculoskeletal health and activities of daily living [17]. Beyond its anatomical role, skeletal muscle serves as a dynamic indicator of health and a key factor in the success of spine medical interventions. As healthcare evolves, prioritizing and understanding spine muscle health will undoubtedly lead to better patient care, improved surgical outcomes in spinal procedures, and a more holistic approach to spinal health management.

1.3 Sarcopenia, frailty and spine pathologies

Frailty and sarcopenia, while interconnected, have different scopes. Frailty refers to the state of decreased physiological reserve, where the body systems no longer maintain a state of homeostasis, ultimately leading to vulnerability to stressors and risk of adverse health outcomes [16, 18]. This multidimensional condition extends beyond physical factors, incorporating psychological, social, and cognitive elements [2, 16, 18]. While often associated with aging, frailty can also result from chronic disease, malnutrition, or other factors that compromise an individual's ability to withstand stressors or maintain normal functioning [18]. Conversely, sarcopenia focuses on muscle loss and weakness, the physical component of frailty [2]. Sarcopenia, situated within the larger framework of frailty, can be used to guide healthcare strategies, including treatment decisions, rehabilitation approaches, and surgical risk assessments for individuals with spine-related pathologies [18]. In the context of spine care, sarcopenia and frailty are crucial considerations as they reflect a decline in health, serving as a predictive indicator for adverse outcomes.

Central to the dynamic between frailty and spine pathologies is the phenomenon of muscle loss, commonly known as sarcopenia. Physiological changes in muscle composition and function become increasingly pronounced with age [3]. These changes collectively contribute to a gradual loss of muscle mass and strength [3]. As muscles weaken, the spine, reliant on muscular support for stability and function, becomes more susceptible to degenerative changes and the development of pathologies [9, 12].

Spine pathologies, ranging from cancer to degenerative disc disease, significantly impact overall health. The localized pain and discomfort are just the tip of the iceberg. Impaired mobility and restrictions in daily activities contribute to a cascade of negative effects on an individual's quality of life, physical and emotional well-being, and overall function [19, 20]. In individuals with spine conditions, sarcopenia acts as a catalyst further exacerbating the challenges they face [20]. The cumulative health consequences highlight the need for a comprehensive approach to spinal health, acknowledging the complex relationship between musculoskeletal health, frailty, and sarcopenia.

Building upon this information, the chapter will provide a comprehensive understanding of the relationship between sarcopenia and spine-related pathologies, including the consequences of sarcopenia, post-treatment/surgical adverse events, various treatments, and the future direction of sarcopenia management in spine-related pathologies.

2. Link between abnormalities in muscle mass and function with the development of spine-related pathologies

The link between abnormalities in muscle mass and function with the development of spine-related pathologies is rooted in the complex relationship between the musculoskeletal system and spinal structures. Muscle mass, a cornerstone of the musculoskeletal system, plays a pivotal role in providing support, stability, and functional mobility to the spine [9]. Skeletal muscles act as dynamic stabilizers, working in concert with ligaments and bones to maintain spine alignment [11]. Changes in muscle mass, commonly observed in conditions like sarcopenia, set the stage for a cascade of musculoskeletal challenges, particularly in the context of spine-related disorders [13]. The complexity of muscle alterations, including atrophy, fatty infiltration, and connective tissue changes, is acknowledged, with the recognition that a single imaging-based biomarker may not be universally applicable [6]. However, the paraspinal and psoas muscles have been heavily implicated in various spinal pathologies [10, 13, 15].

Weak and atrophied muscles struggle to adequately support the spine, placing significant stress on the vertebrae, intervertebral discs, and other spinal structures [21].

The lack of muscular support contributes to the development and progression of spine pathologies including degenerative disc disease, lumbar spinal stenosis, and chronic low back pain [9, 12, 13]. Additionally, muscle groups that are either excessively tight or weak can alter the biomechanics of the spine, leading to postural conditions like lordosis or kyphosis [22]. These postural abnormalities not only compromise the structural integrity of the spine, but also predispose individuals to pain, reduced mobility, and an increased risk of injuries [22]. By addressing the relationship between muscle abnormalities and spine-related pathologies, individuals may prevent the onset of musculoskeletal issues and foster resilience in the face of complex musculoskeletal challenges [14].

3. Consequences of sarcopenia on spine-related pathologies

3.1 Physical function

Sarcopenia can significantly impact physical function in individuals with spine pathologies, increasing the risk of disability, falls, and fractures [1, 4, 5, 23, 24]. Muscle weakness, particularly in the lower back and core muscles, compromises spinal support, leading to postural issues and functional limitations [3, 22]. Functional limitations, such as difficulty walking, lifting objects, and climbing stairs are frequently experienced by those with sarcopenia [3]. Furthermore, the nexus between sarcopenia and decreased bone mineral density significantly increases the risk of fractures, particularly vertebral fractures, among individuals with spine-related pathologies [18]. Additionally, decreased paraspinal muscle mass and strength impair protective reflexes, increasing the risk of fractures, especially vertebral fractures, further affecting physical function [24]. Studies highlight the importance of assessing paraspinal muscle quality in predicting outcomes following spine surgery [25]. These findings highlight the need for targeted exercise interventions, proper nutrition, and comprehensive strategies to address the multifaceted impact of sarcopenia on physical function.

3.2 Psychological factors

Sarcopenia significantly impacts psychological factors in individuals with spine-related pathologies, extending its influence beyond physical health to various aspects of mental well-being. Muscular changes associated with sarcopenia may contribute to increased pain perception and discomfort in individuals with spine pathologies [26]. Heightened pain perception and disability may induce stress and decrease quality of life, independence, and overall well-being, contributing to mental health conditions such as depression and anxiety [3, 5]. Numerous studies emphasize the relationship between psychological factors and sarcopenia in patients with lumbar spinal stenosis and chronic low back pain [27–29]. Thus, healthcare professionals treating spine-related pathologies should consider psychosocial factors such as pain catastrophizing, kinesiophobia, and their influence on pain and disability outcomes [30]. Recognizing and addressing the psychological aspects of sarcopenia in individuals with spine pathology is crucial for providing comprehensive care, promoting mental health, and improving overall health outcomes.

3.3 Quality of life

Sarcopenia, particularly within the context of spine pathology, significantly compromises the quality of life for affected individuals [4]. The consequences of sarcopenia are profound, characterized by functional limitations stemming from muscle loss and weakness, hindering movement and daily activities [4]. The decrease in movement and increase in risks of falls and fractures negatively affect independence and autonomy [1]. Furthermore, chronic pain is exacerbated by sarcopenia, as weakened muscles fail to adequately support the spine leading to increased discomfort and psychological distress, including symptoms of depression and anxiety [4, 12, 13, 24]. Pain may also adversely impact sleep quality, triggering a vicious cycle affecting energy levels, mood, and daily function [31]. Additionally, the economic burden associated with sarcopenia-related complications, such as falls and fractures, increases healthcare use and costs, contributing to stress and further affecting overall quality of life [24]. Studies, such as those by Iwahashi et al. highlight the relationship between sarcopenia, spine pathology, and quality of life, emphasizing the need for comprehensive treatment approaches that address physical, psychological, and social dimensions [26].

4. Linking sarcopenia, spine pathologies, adverse events

4.1 Treatment-related adverse events

Sarcopenia emerges as a critical factor influencing treatment-related adverse events in individuals with spinal pathologies. Studies consistently indicate an elevated risk of moderate to severe treatment-related adverse events in patients with sarcopenia, particularly in the context of spinal cancer, cautioning against postoperative chemotherapy for this population [32, 33]. Notably, low skeletal muscle mass is a significant indicator of incomplete cisplatin-based chemoradiation and dose-limiting toxicities [34]. The relationship between low skeletal muscle mass and toxicity is attributed to the predominant distribution of drugs like cisplatin into the fat-free mass, where skeletal muscle mass is a major contributor [35]. Moreover, cancer patients with sarcopenia report higher rates of pain, nausea, vomiting, dyspnea, insomnia, fatigue, and appetite loss, contributing to a lower overall quality of life [31].

Spine surgery is another prevalent treatment in diverse spinal diseases [9, 12]. Despite efforts to pinpoint potential risk factors associated with complications in spine surgery, only a limited number of prognostic factors have been identified [9]. Back muscle morphometry (i.e., atrophy, fatty infiltration), widely recognized as a prognostic factor in various medical and surgical fields, has garnered attention. In the context of spine surgery, alterations in paraspinal muscle composition are acknowledged contributors to adverse events. Multiple systematic reviews highlight the association between paraspinal muscle health and postoperative outcomes [9, 12]. Increased fatty infiltration and atrophy in the paraspinal muscles (i.e., multifidus, erector spinae) were associated with increased risk of adjacent segment disease or degeneration, proximal junctional kyphosis, sagittal imbalance, pedicle screw loosening, and bone nonunion [12]. In cases where spine surgery is deemed necessary, evaluating paraspinal muscle health before the procedure could serve as an approach to categorizing patients based on their risk of experiencing post-surgical complications [9, 12].

Sarcopenia is also linked to broader treatment-related adverse effects such as physical disability, poor quality of life, falls, fractures, and increased mortality in individuals [23]. These findings reinforce the importance of considering sarcopenia and muscle health in the comprehensive management of individuals with spinal pathologies, particularly when designing treatment strategies.

4.2 Postoperative outcomes

Sarcopenia emerges as a critical factor influencing postoperative outcomes in individuals with spine pathologies undergoing surgical interventions. Studies highlight the potential complications associated with sarcopenia, including delayed recovery, functional decline, increased hospital stay, and rehabilitation difficulty [36–38]. The impact is seen across various surgeries, from emergency laparotomies, lumbar arthrodesis, and spine cancer. In emergency laparotomies, sarcopenia, assessed through skeletal muscle mass index, is linked to poor physiological reserve, perioperative risk, and morbidity in diverse cancer groups [36]. Additionally, the association between sarcopenia and complications after lumbar arthrodesis, such as urinary tract infections and hospital readmissions, coupled with higher complication rates in patients with sarcopenia undergoing surgery for spine cancer, highlights the importance of comprehensive preoperative assessments [39, 40]. Sarcopenia plays a critical role in shaping postoperative outcomes in various spine-related interventions, prompting the need for tailored preoperative strategies to mitigate associated risks.

4.3 Increased mortality

Sarcopenia is associated with increased mortality and adverse outcomes in various spinal-related pathologies. Studies show its independent predictive value for overall survival and recurrence-free survival in cervical spine cancer patients, regardless of treatment modality [41, 42]. Studies evaluating spinal metastasis patients undergoing surgery emphasize the significance of assessing frailty and sarcopenia, with psoas muscle size identified as a robust predictor of both 90-day and overall mortality [43]. Moreover, the assessment of sarcopenia, determined by the third lumbar vertebrae using the total psoas area and vertebral body area on CT scans, proves to be a practical and independent predictor of early postoperative mortality and adverse events in patients with metastatic spinal disease, highlighting its utility in guiding therapeutic decision-making [44]. Additionally, a meta-analysis focusing on spinal metastasis patients reveals a significant association between sarcopenia, assessed through CT scans, and overall survival, reinforcing its role as an indicator of increased mortality risk and a potential guide for treatment decisions [45]. The rising incidence of spinal metastases, affecting approximately 30% of metastatic disease patients, underscores the importance of novel biomarkers like sarcopenia, in predicting mortality and complementing existing prognostic tools for surgical treatment decisions [46].

5. Spine-related sarcopenia treatments

5.1 Importance of tailored treatments

A multidisciplinary and personalized approach to treating spine pathologies and sarcopenia is imperative for optimizing patient outcomes and minimizing potential adverse events [3]. Older age, for instance, may correlate with reduced physiological resilience and an increased susceptibility to treatment-related side effects [3, 14]. Moreover, an advanced clinical stage often indicates a more aggressive disease, mandating tailored therapeutic strategies to address its unique challenges. Conditions like hepatic and renal diseases can impact drug metabolism and clearance, necessitating careful consideration of treatment strategies. Additionally, low socioeconomic status can present barriers to accessing and adhering to care. The identification of contributing factors underscores the importance of a comprehensive assessment that extends beyond the traditional medical parameters. This approach aligns with the paradigm shift towards patient-centered care, recognizing the diverse factors that influence treatment response and overall quality of life.

5.2 Effective rehabilitation strategies

Although research suggests that interventions targeting sarcopenia can significantly improve overall well-being, quality of life, and strength, [23, 47–49], the exploration of effective rehabilitation strategies for sarcopenia in spine-related pathologies remains largely unexplored. While the detrimental impact of sarcopenia on adverse and post-operative outcomes is well-documented, the pre-operative phase offers a potential avenue for interventions to mitigate its effects. The scarcity of comprehensive studies highlights the need for focused research initiatives to develop innovative approaches addressing sarcopenia pre-operatively, ultimately enhancing patient outcomes and quality of care. Drawing from prior research, successful rehabilitation strategies for sarcopenia in spine-related pathologies encompass targeted exercise, nutritional support, and lifestyle modifications [3, 20, 23, 50–53]. Thus, adopting a multidimensional approach emerges as a potentially optimal form of rehabilitation.

5.2.1 Exercise interventions

Individuals with spine-related pain frequently find themselves trapped in a cycle of pain and reduced activity, resulting in deconditioning [3, 54]. Exercise can be a powerful tool to break this cycle. Research demonstrates its effectiveness in improving quality of life, mental health, and pain, irrespective of sarcopenia [47, 55]. Notably, the positive impact of exercise extends to molecular, cellular, and tissue levels, promoting tendon strength, tissue quality during healing, and support for cartilage and bone [56].

Certain types of physical activity, meeting standard levels recommended by the American Heart Association, may not effectively sustain lean mass [20]. However, resistance exercises, involving body weight, free weights (i.e., barbells, dumbbells), or exercise tools (i.e., machines, elastic bands) significantly contribute to musculoskeletal well-being and serve as a preventive measure against sarcopenia, osteoporosis, and the associated risks of falls and fractures [57]. Resistance training and multimodal exercises have demonstrated positive outcomes in addressing spinal sarcopenia by enhancing muscle mass, strength, and overall physical performance [4, 23]. An intervention tailored for elderly women with spinal sarcopenia incorporated back extensor strengthening exercises coupled with protein supplementation [58]. Post-intervention results revealed a significant improvement in physical function, although there were non-significant increases observed in lower extremity muscle mass and back extensor strength. Additionally, numerous studies suggest high-intensity resistance and impact exercise to effectively reduce pain, disability, and gait disturbances while improving lumbar spine bone mineral density, and skeletal muscle mass regardless of sarcopenia [4, 55]. Engaging in high-intensity resistance training produces strain patterns on the bone and yields a significant osteogenic response [55–57]. On the other hand, research suggests that lower-intensity exercise such as walking can be just as effective as other exercise interventions in improving physical quality of life and reducing pain and disability for individuals with chronic low back pain and lumbar cancer [59, 60].

Stabilization and motor control exercises, focusing on deep abdominal muscle activation, have emerged as promising interventions for addressing various spine-related pathologies [13, 61]. Core stabilization and motor control exercises have yielded significant improvements in pain, disability, and lumbar spine paraspinal muscle morphology and function among patients with low back pain [13, 61]. A study comparing core stabilization exercises with strength training exercises in patients with low back pain revealed superior improvements in proprioception, balance, and disability in individuals completing core stabilization exercises [62]. These exercises likely enhance sensory-motor integration and postural control by targeting muscles such as the transversus abdominis and lumbar multifidus [62].

Pilates, a form of exercise emphasizing core strength, flexibility, and body awareness, has gained popularity as a therapeutic option for individuals with spine pathologies. Its focus on core stabilization, spinal alignment, controlled movements, and breathing techniques may alleviate symptoms associated with conditions like low back pain, scoliosis, and lumbar disc herniation [48, 63, 64]. Research suggests that Pilates may effectively address spinal deformities, and improve posture, core stability, pain, function, and quality of life in individuals with spine pathologies [47, 48].

Tai Chi, a traditional Chinese martial art, is increasingly recognized for its potential therapeutic benefits in managing spine pathologies. Research indicates that Tai Chi training leads to significant improvements in muscle strength, endurance, postural balance, and flexibility, particularly in the thoracolumbar spine region [65]. The improvement in pain and disability may be attributed to a decrease in pain catastrophizing [66]. Additionally, individuals who practice Tai Chi have been observed to exhibit fewer degenerative conditions in the lumbar vertebrae and discs, suggesting a potential role in delaying age-related bone loss and strengthening muscles in the lumbar region [67].

Yoga, a mind-body practice, has garnered attention as a therapeutic intervention for various spine pathologies, particularly chronic non-specific low back pain and osteoporosis [68, 69]. Focusing on stability, flexibility, and varied movements (i.e., spine flexion and extension) may alleviate pain, improve posture, strengthen muscles, enhance balance, slow the natural aging process of intervertebral discs, and promote overall spinal health [69, 70]. The holistic approach addresses not only physical symptoms but also psychological well-being, stress reduction, and mindfulness, which are essential components of spine pathology management [71].

While many exercise modes show promise in spine pathology management, further high-quality research is needed to establish protocols for various pathologies and determine whether interventions can elicit significant muscle morphological and functional changes.

5.2.2 Physical therapy

Physical therapy plays a crucial role in the management of spine-related pathologies, offering a comprehensive approach to improving pain, function, and quality of life for patients [72, 73]. Through patient education, manual therapy techniques, modalities (i.e., heat, cold, electrical), and tailored exercises, physical therapists aim to address the underlying causes of spine-related pathologies. These interventions often target posture, range of motion, flexibility, mobility, strength, and endurance to promote healing, target deficiencies, reduce strain on the spine, and prevent future injury. A randomized controlled trial showed significant improvements in symptoms, function, walking distance, pain, disability, and physical activity for patients with lumbar spine stenosis receiving frequent supervised physical therapy sessions [72]. Equipping patients with knowledge and the right tools through physical therapy empowers them to actively participate in their recovery and improve spinal health.

5.2.3 Complementary medicine

Massage therapy may offer benefits in reducing pain and improving function in spine-related pathologies. A review suggested short-term benefits for acute and subacute pain and disability, but effects on chronic pain were mixed, with it being less effective than manipulative therapy in some studies [74]. The precise mechanisms underlying the therapeutic effects of massage therapy on spine pathologies are not fully understood but its role in promoting relaxation and circulation likely plays a significant role. Acupuncture offers similar benefits, providing short-term pain relief and improving disability for chronic neck pain, low back pain, and even osteoporosis [75, 76]. Studies on acupuncture for osteoporosis suggest positive effects on bone quality and symptom reduction [76]. Preliminary evidence from animal research points towards potential mechanisms for acupuncture, including its impact on hormone levels, inflammatory responses, and bone-related signaling pathways. However, challenges remain in translating these findings to clinical practice and fully understanding the molecular mechanisms. Manipulations and mobilizations for spine pathologies reveal varying degrees of effectiveness and safety. While a systematic review and meta-analysis revealed spinal manipulative interventions significantly reduced pain and disability in chronic low back pain [77], another review yielded mixed results, indicating benefits in some cases, but no differences in others [78]. Though promising for managing spine-related pathologies, complementary medicine requires further research to optimize treatment protocols and solidify effectiveness.

5.2.4 Nutritional interventions

Nutritional interventions play a crucial role in addressing sarcopenia in spine-related pathologies, offering promising avenues for treatment [4]. A narrative review by Candow et al. emphasized the potential of creatine monohydrate supplementation, particularly when combined with resistance training, as an effective treatment for sarcopenia and related conditions in older adults [50]. The review suggests that creatine, when used in conjunction with resistance training, exhibits favorable effects on aging muscle and bone, positioning it as a promising intervention for sarcopenia, frailty, and cachexia. Vitamin D, as explored by Haeri et al., has been associated with positive outcomes for bone microarchitecture and gait speed in older women with osteoporosis [51]. The study indicates a significant positive correlation between vitamin D levels and spine trabecular bone, as well as gait speed. This suggests that maintaining adequate vitamin D levels is linked to improved bone health and physical function, showcasing the potential of nutritional strategies in managing sarcopenia in the context of osteoporosis. Furthermore, a systematic review by Abdelhamid et al. investigated the effects of dietary omega-3 and omega-6 polyunsaturated fatty acids on musculoskeletal outcomes and functional status in adults over the age of 40 [52]. While the evidence is limited, omega-3 is suggested to have protective effects on bone and muscle, whereas omega-6 may have pro-inflammatory effects detrimental to musculoskeletal health. The review underscores the importance of understanding how nutritional factors, including fatty acids, contribute to musculoskeletal health during aging. In a different context, examining dietary patterns in patients with gastrointestinal cancer, Velho et al. identified a dietary pattern high in fat and fish associated with reduced odds of sarcopenia [53]. This suggests that specific dietary choices may impact the development of sarcopenia, emphasizing the role of nutrition in mitigating the condition. Studies also suggest that antioxidants such as resveratrol, β-hydroxy-β-methyl butyrate, and green tea catechins can improve satellite cell functions during rehabilitative loading after disuse, further emphasizing the role of nutrition in preserving musculoskeletal health [20]. This evidence collectively underscores the significance of tailored nutritional interventions as part of a multidimensional approach to managing sarcopenia in spine-related pathologies.

5.2.5 Pharmacological interventions

The management of sarcopenia in spine-related pathologies may involve exploring pharmacological interventions [4, 79]. Current recommendations primarily rely on physical activity and nutritional interventions, leaving a critical gap in addressing sarcopenia within spine-related conditions pharmacologically [79]. The urgency to develop new drugs capable of restoring both muscle mass and function is emphasized by the limited success of existing approaches. Trials have investigated selective androgen receptor modulators, myostatin antibodies, and other agents, yet their clinical efficacy remains unclear [20]. Additionally, pharmacological interventions for spine-related conditions, such as degenerative disc diseases and osteoporosis, present challenges. The use of nonsteroidal anti-inflammatory drugs (NSAIDs) and benzodiazepines for back pain and degenerative disc disease may offer pain relief, but surgery becomes necessary in severe cases, bringing its own set of challenges [79]. Osteoporosis, on the other hand, is primarily managed with bisphosphonates, although their long-term use is limited by significant side effects [79]. Despite advancements, the current pharmacological field faces obstacles, necessitating ongoing research and the development of novel therapies to address the complex nature of spine-related pathologies comprehensively.

5.2.6 Regenerative approach

Recent advancements in regenerative approaches for treating spinal sarcopenia involve innovative strategies such as stem-cell-based therapies, biological scaffolds, and platelet-rich plasma. Stem-cell-based strategies, as explored in animal studies, encompass the use of various cell types, including satellite cells, muscle-derived stem cells, and embryonic stem cells, to address skeletal muscle repair [20]. Preclinical studies have shown the promising potential of stem cell-based therapies, specifically those involving muscle-derived stem cells, in enhancing muscle repair, positioning them as a viable option for treating spinal sarcopenia. Biological scaffolds, composed of mammalian extracellular matrix, offer a promising therapeutic option by preserving skeletal muscle function and preventing spinal sarcopenia [20]. This approach aids in site-appropriate remodeling of skeletal muscle, correcting myofiber alignment and maintaining mechanical properties crucial for tissue function. Additionally, platelet-rich plasma shows promise in modulating molecular factors crucial for effective muscle injury repair and regeneration [20]. While these regenerative approaches hold potential, further research, particularly human trials, is essential to fully comprehend their effectiveness in managing spinal sarcopenia.

6. Comprehensive approach

Spine care providers, through a comprehensive approach that spans both non-operative and operative care strategies, acknowledge the diverse nature of spinal pathologies and the need for tailored interventions. The integration of Enhanced Recovery After Surgery (eRAS) protocols seamlessly aligns with this comprehensive perspective, constituting an interdisciplinary strategy to elevate patient care by integrating evidence-based methodologies from pre-operation to post-operation [80]. The interventions embedded in eRAS protocols are grounded in the fundamental principle that patient outcomes can be substantially enhanced by effectively managing pain, promoting early ambulation, attending physical therapy, and addressing nutritional needs to prevent catabolism and immune dysfunction. By addressing not only the physical manifestations of spine-related pathologies but also considering patient-reported quality of life and potential adverse events, spine care providers elevate the standard of care while striving for cost-effective solutions without compromising efficacy.

7. Future research

Addressing the relationship between skeletal muscle morphology, function, and spinal pathologies opens promising avenues for future research. Exploring the role of exercise modalities, nutritional interventions, and emerging therapeutics in preserving muscle health and improving spinal pathologies presents a promising path forward. Identifying potential treatment and prevention strategies based on evidence-based findings could revolutionize clinical approaches, offering novel interventions aimed at mitigating the impact of sarcopenia on spine health and improving the quality of life for individuals affected by these conditions. This perspective will not only enrich the current understanding of sarcopenia, musculoskeletal health and spine-related pathologies, but also foster innovation and guide future advancements in the field of musculoskeletal health.

8. Conclusions

The intricate relationship between sarcopenia and spine pathologies unveils a multifaceted impact that extends beyond mere musculoskeletal concerns. From compromised spinal stability to diminished bone density, the consequences of sarcopenia reverberate through the intricate biomechanics of the spine. Sarcopenia serves not only as a diagnostic tool but also as a modifiable variable, playing a pivotal role in shaping pre-operative, non-operative care, and post-operative outcomes, as well as influencing rehabilitation strategies. The relationship between muscle loss, spinal health, adverse events, and quality of life highlights the need for a comprehensive approach that encompasses research, healthcare, and public health initiatives to manage and prevent these conditions. As the healthcare industry strives for a comprehensive understanding of the complex connection between sarcopenia and spine pathologies, interventions addressing biological, psychological, and social elements are crucial in mitigating the impact and improving the overall quality of life for individuals grappling with these health challenges.

Conflict of interest

The authors declare no conflict of interest.

Author details

Chanelle Montpetit[1], Michael H. Weber[2] and Maryse Fortin[1]*

1 Department of Health, Kinesiology and Applied Physiology, Concordia University, Montreal, Quebec, Canada

2 Spine Surgery Program, Department of Surgery, McGill University, Montreal, Canada

*Address all correspondence to: maryse.fortin@concordia.ca

References

[1] Santilli V, Bernetti A, Mangone M, Paoloni M. Clinical definition of sarcopenia. Clinical Cases in Mineral and Bone Metabolism. 2014;**11**(3):177-180

[2] Cruz-Jentoft AJ, Bahat G, Bauer J, Boirie Y, Bruyère O, Cederholm T, et al. Sarcopenia: Revised European consensus on definition and diagnosis. Age and Ageing. 2019;**48**(1):16-31. DOI: 10.1093/ageing/afy169

[3] Park WT, Shon OJ, Kim GB. Multidisciplinary approach to sarcopenia: A narrative review. Journal of Yeungnam Medical Science. 2023;**40**(4):352-363. DOI: 10.12701/jyms.2023.00724

[4] Papadopoulou SK. Sarcopenia: A contemporary health program among older adult populations. Nutrients. 2020;**12**(5):1293. DOI: 10.3390/nu12051293

[5] Beaudart C, Rizzoli R, Bruyère O, Reginster JY, Biver E. Sarcopenia: Burden and challenges for public health. Archives of Public Health. 2014;**72**:45. DOI: 10.1186/2049-3258-72-45

[6] Hodges PW, Bailey JF, Fortin M, Battié MC. Paraspinal muscle imaging measurements for common spinal disorders: Review and consensus-based recommendations from the ISSLS degenerative spinal phenotypes group. European Spine Journal. 2021;**30**:3428-3441. DOI: 10.1007/s00586-021-06990-2

[7] van de Velde NM, Koeks Z, Signorelli M, Verwey N, Overzier M, Bakker JA, et al. Longitudinal assessment of creatine kinase, creatine/creatinine ratio, and myostatin as monitoring biomarkers in Becker Muscular Dystrophy. Neurology. 2023;**100**(9):e975-e984. DOI: 10.1212/WNL.0000000000201609

[8] Moon JH, Kim KM, Kim JH, Moon JH, Choi SH, Lim S, et al. Predictive values of the new sarcopenia index by the foundation for the National Institutes of Health sarcopenia project for mortality among older Korean adults. PLoS One. 2016;**11**(11):e0166344. DOI: 10.1371/journal.pone.0166344

[9] Khan AB, Weiss EH, Khan AW, Omeis I, Verla T. Back muscle morphometry: Effects on outcomes of spine surgery. World Neurosurgery. 2017;**103**:174-179. DOI: 10.1016/j.wneu.2017.03.097

[10] Frontera WR, Ochala J. Skeletal muscle: A brief review of structure and function. Calcified Tissue International. 2015;**96**:183-195. DOI: 10.1007/s00223-014-9915-y

[11] Gibbons D, McDonnell JM, Ahern DP, Cunniffe G, Kenny RA, Romero-Ortuno R, et al. The relationship between radiological paraspinal lumbar measures and clinical measures of sarcopenia in older adults with chronic lower back pain. Journal of Frailty, Sarcopenia and Falls. 2022;7(2):52-59. DOI: 10.22540/JFSF-07-052

[12] Gengyu H, Jingyue D, Chunjie G, Bo Z, Yu J, Jiaming L, et al. The predictive value of preoperative paraspinal muscle morphometry on complications after lumbar surgery: A systematic review. European Spine Journal. 2022;**31**:364-379. DOI: 10.1007/s00586-021-07052-3

[13] Fortin M, Rye M, Roussac A, Montpetit C, Burdick J, Nadghi N, et al. The effects of combined motor control and isolated extensor strengthening

versus general exercise on paraspinal muscle morphology, composition, and function in patients with chronic low back pain: A randomized controlled trial. Journal of Clinical Medicine. 2023;**12**(18):5920. DOI: 10.1186/s12891-021-04346-x

[14] Aversa Z, Zhang X, Fielding RA, Lanza I, LeBrasseur NK. The clinical impact and biological mechanisms of skeletal muscle aging. Bone. 2020;**127**:26-36. DOI: 10.1016/j.bone.2019.05.021

[15] Fortin M, Dobrescu O, Courtemanche M, Sparrey CJ, Santaguida C, Fehlings G, et al. Association between paraspinal muscle morphology, clinical symptoms, and functional status in patients with degenerative cervical myelopathy. Spine. 2017;**42**(4):232-239. DOI: 10.1097/BRS.0000000000001704

[16] Guo K, Wang X, Lu X, Yang Y, Lu W, Wensi L, et al. Effects of sarcopenia and frailty on postoperative recovery in elderly patients: A prospective cohort study. Journal of Cachexia, Sarcopenia and Muscle. 2023;**14**(6):2642-2652. DOI: 10.1002/jcsm.13337

[17] Deng D, Lian Z, Cui W, Liang H, Xiao L, Yao G. Function of low back muscle exercise: Preventive effect of refracture analysis of postoperative vertebral fractures. Orthopade. 2019;**48**(4):337-342. DOI: 10.1007/s00132-018-3577-9

[18] Marques A, Queirós C, Santy-Tomlinson J. Frailty and sarcopenia. In: Fragility Fracture and Orthogeriatric Nursing. 2nd ed. Cham: Springer; 2023. pp. 35-52. DOI: 10.1007/978-3-031-33484-9

[19] Makris UE, Higashi RT, Marks EG, Fraenkel L, Gill TM, Friedly JL, et al. Physical, emotional and social impacts of restricting back pain in older adults: A qualitative study. Pain Medicine. 2017;**18**(7):1225-1235. DOI: 10.1093/pm/pnw196

[20] Kuo YK, Lin YC, Lee CY, Chen CY, Tani J, Huang TJ, et al. Novel insights into the pathogenesis of spinal sarcopenia and related therapeutic approaches: A narrative review. International Journal of Molecular Sciences. 2020;**21**(8):3010. DOI: 10.3390/ijms21083010

[21] Sun D, Liu P, Cheng J, Ma Z, Liu J, Qin T. Correlation between intervertebral disc degeneration, paraspinal muscle atrophy, lumbar facet joints degeneration in patients with lumbar disc herniation. BMC Musculoskeletal Disorder. 2017;**18**:167. DOI: 10.1186/s12891-017-1522-4

[22] Singla D, Veqar Z. Association between forward head, rounded shoulders, and increased thoracic kyphosis: A review of the literature. Journal of Chiropractic Medicine. 2017;**16**(3):220-229. DOI: 10.1016/j.jcm.2017.03.004

[23] Tsekoura M, Billis E, Kastrinis A, Katsoulaki M, Fousekis K, Tsepis E, et al. The effects of exercise in patients with sarcopenia. Advances in Experimental Medicine and Biology. 2020;**1337**:251-290. DOI: 10.1007/978-3-030-78771-4_31

[24] Lee DG, Bae JH. Fatty infiltration of the multifidus muscle independently increases osteoporotic vertebral compression fracture risk. BMC Musculoskeletal Disorders. 2023;**24**:508. DOI: 10.1186/s12891-023-06640-2

[25] Zavras AG, Sullivan TB, Federico VP, Nolte MT, Munim MA, Phillips FM, et al. Preoperative multifidus muscle quality is associated with patient reported outcomes after lateral lumbar interbody fusion. Global

Spine Journal. 2024;**14**:647-656. DOI: 10.1177/21925682221120400

[26] Iwahashi S, Hashida R, Matsuse H, Higashi E, Bekki M, Iwanaga S, et al. The impact of sarcopenia on low back pain and quality of life in patients with osteoporosis. BMC Musculoskeletal Disorders. 2022;**23**:142. DOI: 10.1186/s12891-022-05086-2

[27] Wada T, Tanishima S, Osaki M, Nagashima H, Hagino H. Relationship between sarcopenia and pain catastrophizing in patients with lumbar spine stenosis: A cross-sectional study. Osteoporosis and Sarcopenia. 2019;**5**(4):132-136. DOI: 10.1016/j.afos.2019.12.001

[28] Wada T, Tanishima S, KitsudaY,OsakiM,NagashimaH,HaginoH. Association between preoperative low muscle mass and psychological factors after surgery among patients with lumbar spine stenosis: A longitudinal study. Journal of Clinical Neuroscience. 2021;**89**:8-14. DOI: 10.1016/j.jocn.2021.04.008

[29] Jadhakhan F, Sobeih R, Falla D. Effects of exercise/physical activity on fear of movement in people with spine-related pain: A systematic review. Frontiers in Psychology. 2023;**14**:1213199. DOI: 10.3389/fpsyg.2023.1213199

[30] Alhowimel A, AlOtaibi M, Radford K, Coulson N. Psychosocial factors associated with change in pain and disability outcomes in chronic low back pain patients treated by physiotherapist: A systematic review. SAGE Open Medicine. 2018;**6**:2050312118757387. DOI: 10.1177/2050312118757387

[31] Finan PH, Goodin BR, Smith MT. The association of sleep and pain: An update and a path forward. Journal of Pain. 2014;**14**(12):1539-1552. DOI: 10.1016/j.jpain.2013.08.007

[32] Vergara N, Montoya JE, Lunda HG, Amparo JR, Cristal-Luna G. Quality of life and nutritional status among cancer patients on chemotherapy. Oman Medical Journal. 2013;**28**(4):270-274. DOI: 10.5001/omj.2013.75

[33] Tan BHL, Brammer K, Randhawa N, Welch NT, Parsons SL, James EJ, et al. Sarcopenia is associated with toxicity in patients undergoing neo-adjuvant chemotherapy for oesophago-gastric cancer. European Journal of Surgical Oncology. 2015;**41**(3):333-338. DOI: 10.1016/j.ejso.2014.11.040

[34] Wendrich AW, Swartz JE, Bril SI, Wegner I, de Graeff A, Smid EJ, et al. Low skeletal muscle mass is a predictive factor for chemotherapy dose-limiting toxicity in patients with locally advanced head and neck cancer. Oral Oncology. 2017;**71**:26-33. DOI: 10.1016/j.oraloncology.2017.05.012

[35] de Bree R, Meerkerk CDA, Halmos GB, Mäkitie AA, Homma A, Rodrigo JP, et al. Measurement of sarcopenia in head and neck cancer patients and its association with frailty. Frontiers in Oncology. 2022;**12**:884988. DOI: 10.3389/fonc.2022.884988

[36] Body S, Ligthart MAP, Rahman S, Ward J, May-Miller P, Pucher PH, et al. Sarcopenia and Myosteatosis predict adverse outcomes after emergency laparotomy. Annals of Surgery. 2022;**275**(6):1103-1111. DOI: 10.1097/SLA.0000000000004781

[37] Pinter ZW, Salmons HI, Townsley S, Omar A, Freedman BA, Currier BL, et al. Multifidus sarcopenia is associated with worse patient-reported

outcomes following posterior cervical decompression and fusion. Spine. 2022;**47**(20):1426-1434. DOI: 10.1097/BRS.0000000000004386

[38] Bokshan SL, Han AL, DePasse JM, Eltorai AEM, Maracaccio SE, Palumbo MA, et al. Effect of sarcopenia on postoperative morbidity and mortality after thoracolumbar spine surgery. Orthopedics. 2016;**39**(6):e1159-e1164. DOI: 10.3928/01477447-20160811-02

[39] Jung AR, Roh JL, Kim JS, Choi SH, Nam SY, Kim SY. The impact of skeletal muscle depletion in older adult patients with head and neck cancer undergoing primary surgery. Journal of Geriatric Oncology. 2021;**12**:128-133. DOI: 10.1016/j.jgo.2020.06.009

[40] Albright JA, Chang K, Alsoof D, McDonald CL, Diebo BG, Daniels AH. Sarcopenia and postoperative complications, cost of care, and all-cause hospital readmission following lumbar spine arthrodesis: A propensity matched cohort study. World Neurosurgery. 2023;**169**:e131-e140. DOI: 10.1016/j.wneu.2022.10.077

[41] McCabe FJ, McCabe JP, Murray O. A novel scoring system incorporating sarcopenia to predict postoperative survival in spinal metastasis. The Spine Journal. 2023;**23**(9):1270-1275. DOI: 10.1016/j.spinee.2023.04.010

[42] Jovanovic N, Chinnery T, Mattonen SA, Palma DA, Doyle PC, Theurer JA. Sarcopenia in head and neck cancer: A scoping review. PLoS One. 2022;**17**(11):1-24. DOI: 10.1371/journal.pone.0278135

[43] Zakaria HS, Wilkinson BM, Pennington Z, Saadeh YS, Lau D, Chandra A, et al. Sarcopenia as a prognostic factor for 90-day and overall mortality in patients undergoing spine surgery for metastatic tumors: A multicenter retrospective cohort study. Neurosurgery. 2020;**87**(5):1025-1036. DOI: 10.1093/neuros/nyaa245

[44] Bourassa-Moreau E, Versteeg A, Moskven E, Charest-Morin R, Flexman A, Ailon T, et al. Sarcopenia, but not frailty, predicts early mortality and adverse events after emergent surgery for metastatic disease of the spine. The Spine Journal. 2020;**20**(1):22-31. DOI: 10.1016/j.spinee.2019.08.012

[45] Tan H, Gao X, Li X, Huang Y, Cao Q, Wan T. Sarcopenia in patients with spinal metastasis: A systematic review and meta-analysis of retrospective cohort studies. Frontiers in Oncology. 2022;**12**:864501. DOI: 10.3389/fonc.2022.864501

[46] Bongers MER, Groot OQ, Buckless CG, Kapoor ND, Twining PK, Schwab JH, et al. Body composition predictors of mortality on CT in patients with spinal metastases undergoing surgical treatment. The Spine Journal. 2022;**22**(4):595-604. DOI: 10.1016/j.spinee.2021.10.011

[47] Schwartz CE, Stark RB, Balasuberamaniam P, Shrikumar M, Wasim A, Finkelstein JA. Moving toward better health: Exercise practice is associated with improved outcomes after spine surgery in people with degenerative lumbar conditions. Canadian Journal of Surgery. 2021;**64**(4):E419-E427. DOI: 10.1503/cjs.010620

[48] Li F, Dev Omar Dev R, Soh KG, Wang C, Yuan Y. Effects of pilates exercises on spine deformities and posture: A systematic review. BMC Sports Science, Medicine and Rehabilitation. 2024;**16**:55. DOI: 10.1186/s13102-024-00843-3

[49] Shi J, Hu ZY, Wen YR, Wang YF, Lin YY, Zhao HZ, et al. Optimal modes of mind-body exercise for treating chronic non-specific low back pain: Systematic review and network meta-analysis. Frontiers in Neuroscience. 2022;**16**:1046518. DOI: 10.3389/fnins.2022.1046518

[50] Candow DG, Chilibeck PD, Forbes SC, Fairman CM, Gualano B, Roschel H. Creatine supplementation for older adults: Focus on sarcopenia, osteoporosis, frailty and cachexia. Bone. 2022;**162**:116467. DOI: 10.1016/j.bone.2022.116467

[51] Haeri NS, Perera S, Greenspan SL. The association of vitamin D with bone microarchitecture, muscle strength, and mobility performance in older women in long-term care. Bone. 2023;**176**:116867. DOI: 10.1016/j.bone.2023.116867

[52] Abdelhamid A, Hooper L, Sivakaran R, Hayhoe RPG, Welch A. The relationship between Omega-3, Omega-6 and total polyunsaturated fat and musculoskeletal health and functional status in adults: A systematic review and meta-analysis of RCTs. Calcified Tissue International. 2019;**105**:353-372. DOI: 10.1007/s00223-019-00584-3

[53] Velho S, Moço S, Ferreira A, Cruz R, Agostinho L, Cabral MS, et al. Dietary patterns and their relationship to sarcopenia in Portuguese patients with gastrointestinal cancer: An exploratory study. Nutrition. 2019;**63**(64):193-199. DOI: 10.1016/j.nut.2019.01.014

[54] Linton SJ, Shaw WS. Impact of psychological factors in the experience of pain. Physical Therapy. 2011;**91**(5):700-711. DOI: 10.2522/ptj.20100330

[55] Kemmler W, Kohl M, Jakob F, Engelke K, von Stengel S. Effects of high intensity dynamic resistance exercise and whey protein supplements on osteosarcopenia in older men with low bone and muscle mass. Final results of the randomized controlled FrOST study. Nutrients. 2020;**12**(8):2341. DOI: 10.3390/nu12082341

[56] Lewis R, Álvarez CBG, Rayman M, Lanham-New S, Woolf A, Mobasheri A. Strategies for optimizing musculoskeletal health in the 21st century. BMC Musculoskeletal Disorders. 2019;**20**:164. DOI: 10.1186/s12891-019-2510-7

[57] Hong AR, Kim SW. Effects of resistance exercise on bone health. Endocrinology Metabolism. 2018;**33**(4):435-444. DOI: 10.3803/EnM.2018.33.4.435

[58] Kim S, Park J, Kim DH, Sun J, Lee SL. Combined exercise and nutrition intervention for older women with spinal sarcopenia: An open-label single-arm trial. BMC Geriatrics. 2023;**23**:346. DOI: 10.1186/s12877-023-04063-1

[59] Zhou Y, Cartmel B, Gottlieb L, Ercolano EA, Li F, Harrigan M, et al. Randomized trial of exercise on quality of life in women with ovarian cancer: Women's activity and lifestyle study in Connecticut (WALC). Journal of National Cancer Institute. 2017;**109**(12):djx072. DOI: 10.1093/jnci/djx072

[60] Sitthipornvorakul E, Klinsophon T, Sihawong R, Janwantanakul P. The effects of walking intervention in patients with chronic low back pain: A meta-analysis of randomized controlled trials. Musculoskeletal Science and Practice. 2018;**34**:38-46. DOI: 10.1016/j.msksp.2017.12.003

[61] Smrcina Z, Woelfel S, Burcal C. A systematic review of the effectiveness of core stability exercises in patients with non-specific low back pain.

International Journal of Sports Physical Therapy. 2022;**17**(5):766-774. DOI: 10.26603/001c.37251

[62] Hlaing SS, Puntumetakul R, Khine EE, Boucaut R. Effects of core stabilization exercise and strengthening exercise on proprioception, balance, muscle thickness and pain related outcomes in patients with subacute nonspecific low back pain: A randomized controlled trial. BMC Musculoskeletal Disorders. 2021;**22**:998. DOI: 10.1186/s12891-021-04858-6

[63] Taşpinar G, Angin E, Oksüz S. The effects of pilates on pain, functionality, quality of life, flexibility and endurance in lumbar disc herniation. Journal of Comparative Effectiveness Research. 2023;**12**(1):e220144. DOI: 10.2217/cer-2022-0144

[64] Çolak TK, Akçay B, Apti A. Effects of pilates exercises on idiopathic scoliosis: A scoping review of the literature. Spine Deformity. 2023;**11**:797-804. DOI: 10.1007/s43390-023-00668-z

[65] Wehner C, Blank C, Arvandi M, Wehner C, Schobersberger W. Effect of Tai Chi on muscle strength, physical endurance, postural balance and flexibility: A systematic review and meta-analysis. BMJ Open Sport & Exercise Medicine. 2021;7(1):e000817. DOI: 10.1136/bmjsem-2020-000817

[66] Hall AM, Kamper SJ, Emsley R, Maher CG. Does pain-catastrophising mediate the effect of tai chi on treatment outcomes for people with low back pain? Complementary Therapies in Medicine. 2016;**25**:61-66. DOI: 10.1016/j.ctim.2015.12.013

[67] Deng C, Xia W. Effect of Tai Chi Chuan on degeneration of lumbar vertebrae and lumbar discs in middle-aged and aged people: A cross-sectional study based on magnetic resonance images. Journal of International Medical Research. 2018;**46**(2):578-585. DOI: 10.1177/0300060517734115

[68] Wieland LS, Santesso N. A summary of a Cochrane review: Yoga treatment for chronic non-specific low back pain. European Journal of Integrative Medicine. 2017;**11**:39-40. DOI: 10.1016/j.eujim.2017.03.003

[69] Smith EN, Boser A. Yoga, vertebral fractures, and osteoporosis: Research and recommendations. International Journal of Yoga Therapy. 2013;**23**(1):17-23

[70] Jeng CM, Cheng TC, Kung CH, Hsu HC. Yoga and disc degenerative disease in cervical and lumbar spine: An MR imaging-based case control study. European Spine Journal. 2011;**20**(3):408-413. DOI: 10.1007/s00586-010-1547-y

[71] Kuvačić G, Fratini P, Padulo J, Iacono AD, De Giorgio A. Effectiveness of yoga and educational intervention on disability, anxiety, depression, and pain in people with CLBP: A randomized controlled trial. Complementary Therapies in Clinical Practice. 2018;**31**:262-267. DOI: 10.1016/j.ctcp.2018.03.008

[72] Minetama M, Kawakami M, Teraguchi M, Kagotani R, Mera Y, Sumiya T, et al. Supervised physical therapy vs. home exercise for patients with lumbar spinal stenosis: A randomized controlled trial. The Spine Journal. 2019;**19**(8):1310-1318. DOI: 10.1016/j.spinee.2019.04.009

[73] Rizzo A. The role of exercise and rehabilitation in the cancer care plan. Journal of Advanced Practitioner in Oncology. 2016;7(3):339-342. DOI: 10.6004/jadpro.2016.7.3.20

[74] Kumar S, Beaton K, Hughes T. The effectiveness of massage therapy for

the treatment of nonspecific low back pain: A systematic review of systematic reviews. International Journal of General Medicine. 2013;**6**:733-741. DOI: 10.2147/IJGM.S50243

[75] Huang JF, Zheng XQ, Chen D, Lin JL, Zhou WX, Wang H, et al. Can acupuncture improve chronic spinal pain? A systematic review and meta-analysis. Global Spine Journal. 2021;**11**(8):1248-1265. DOI: 10.1177/2192568220962440

[76] Tian Y, Wang L, Xu T, Li R, Zhu R, Chen B, et al. Acupuncture for osteoporosis: A review of its clinical and preclinical studies. Journal of Acupuncture & Meridian Studies. 2021;**15**(5):281-299. DOI: 10.51507/j.jams.2022.15.5.281

[77] Coulter ID, Crawford C, Hurwitz EL, Vernon H, Khorsan R, Booth MS, et al. Manipulation and mobilization for treating chronic low back pain: A systematic review and meta-analysis. The Spine Journal. 2018;**18**(5):866-879. DOI: 10.1016/j.spinee.2018.01.013

[78] Gevers-Montoro C, Provencher B, Descarreaux M, Ortega de Mues A. Clinical effectiveness and efficacy of chiropractic spinal manipulation for spine pain. Frontiers in pain. Research. 2021;**2**:865921. DOI: 10.3389/fpain.2021.765921

[79] Yin P, Jiang Y, Fang X, Wang D, Li Y, Chen M, et al. Cell-based therapies for degenerative musculoskeletal diseases. Advanced Science. 2023;**10**(21):2207050. DOI: 10.1002/advs.202207050

[80] Naftalovich R, Singal A, Iskander AJ. Enhanced recovery after surgery (ERAS) protocols for spine surgery – Review of literature. Anesthesiology Intensive Therapy. 2022;**54**(1):71-79. DOI: 10.5114/ait.2022.113961

Chapter 3

Perspective Chapter: Chronic Kidney Disease–Related Sarcopenia Diagnosis in Patients undergoing Hemodialysis

Santiago David Silva Tobar and Leticia Andreina Lozada Tobar

Abstract

Sarcopenia syndrome is a muscle disease characterized by the loss of muscle mass and quality, according to the European Working Group on Sarcopenia in Older People (EWGSOP). In the general population, sarcopenia is closely associated with aging, reduced quality of life, and increased mortality, conditions that aggregate to chronic kidney disease (CKD) and hemodialysis treatment. Sarcopenia and kidney disease wasting (KDW) syndrome are correlated by an interaction of genetic, mechanical, hormonal, inflammatory, and nutritional factors that injure the metabolic muscular system, resulting in cachexia, a severe form of protein-energy wasting. The aim of this review is to comprehensively examine the concept, pathophysiology, and diagnostic criteria of sarcopenia as it pertains to patients with CKD and those undergoing hemodialysis. In this review, we analyzed the diagnosis and physiopathology of chronic kidney disease–related sarcopenia (CKD-RS) in patients undergoing hemodialysis.

Keywords: sarcopenia, frailty, chronic kidney disease, hemodialysis patients, end-stage renal disease

1. Introduction

The aim of this review is to analyze the diagnosis and physiopathology of sarcopenia related to chronic kidney disease (CKD) in patients undergoing hemodialysis.

CKD is a syndrome characterized by uremic symptoms and alterations in the laboratory analyses due to abnormalities of kidney structure or/and function (estimated glomerular filtration rate < 60 ml/min/1.73m^2), present for a time > 3 months, according to the definition of Kidney Disease: Improving Global Outcomes (KDIGO) guidelines [1].

Sarcopenia is defined by the European Working Group on Sarcopenia in Older People 2 (EWGSOP2 in 2018) as a progressive skeletal muscle disorder that impairs muscle function (quality) and mass (quantity) predisposing patients to a major likelihood of falls, fractures, physical disability, and mortality [2–5].

Due to the high prevalence of muscle wasting, malnutrition, and inflammation in CKD and hemodialysis patients, sarcopenia is commonly correlated with kidney disease wasting (KDW) syndrome, characterized by a loss of body protein mass and fuel reserves in CKD patients [2].

Sarcopenia and KDW syndrome are correlated by an interaction of genetic, mechanical, hormonal, inflammatory, and nutritional factors that injure the metabolic muscular system, resulting in cachexia, a severe form of protein-energy wasting (PEW) [2, 3].

Patients, with CKD in any stage included in hemodialysis, have some grade of sarcopenia that in combination with aging, multiple comorbidities, catabolic uremic state, dietary restrictions, and reduced functional capacity generates major mortality in relation to the general population without CKD or hemodialysis [3].

Diagnosis and classification of sarcopenia in the general population, CKD, and hemodialysis patients are based on the clinical characteristics of this syndrome: analysis of decreased muscle strength (muscle failure) with handgrip method, a score of muscle quantity (muscle mass) or quality, and altered tests of physical performance [3, 4].

In the last year, some studies have developed a sarcopenia risk prediction scheme in patients undergoing and in hemodialysis for early identification and timely intervention in high-risk groups based on points according to age, C-reactive protein, body mass index, mid-upper arm muscle circumference, and serum phosphorus levels. However, more studies are necessary for validation in CKD and hemodialysis patients.

2. Epidemiology

A meta-analysis that included cross-sectional or cohort studies of North and South American, European, African, Asian, and Australian participants including 692.056 non-CKD participants with a mean age of 68 years and using a different score of diagnosis and classifications of sarcopenia (Asian Working Group for Sarcopenia, EWGSOP, Foundation for the National Institute of Health, and International Working Group on Sarcopenia) demonstrated a prevalence of sarcopenia in the general population to be between 10 and 27% [6].

A systematic review and meta-analysis with observational and cohort studies of Asia and Europe, including 58.404 non-CKD individuals aged ≥ 60 years, using the EWGSOP score, demonstrate a prevalence of 10% (95% CI: 8–12%) in men and 10% (95% CI: 8–13%) in women [7].

A cross-sectional study determined that a prevalence of sarcopenia in 76 Beijing Jishuitan Hospital patients of 18 years or more undergoing hemodialysis treatment was between 28.5% and 40.3% and was associated with poor outcomes [8]. Sarcopenia was determined by handgrip strength method (HGS), short physical performance battery (SPPB) performance, and appendicular skeletal muscle mass index (ASMI) [8].

The same study demonstrated that the risk factors associated with the apparition of sarcopenia were older age (OR: 1.061, $P < 0.003$); lower body mass index (BMI) (OR: 0.837, $P = 0.008$), albumin (OR: 0.765, $P = 0.004$), prealbumin (OR: 0.987, $P = 0.001$), predialysis blood urea nitrogen (BUN) (OR: 0.842, $P < 0.001$), predialysis creatinine (OR: 0.993, $P < 0.001$), and phosphorus (OR: 0.396, $P = 0.047$); and lower CSA of the thigh (OR: 0.58, $P = 0.035$), third lumbar (L3) trunk (OR: 0.37,

P = 0.004), gluteus minimus and medius (OR: 0.28, P = 0.001), and gluteus maximus (OR: 0.28, P = 0.001) [8, 9].

According to these principal studies, prevalence of sarcopenia in hemodialysis patients is higher than that in the general population without hemodialysis (two times higher approximately). It is frequent in ages >60 years and has no difference with sex.

Some comparative studies indicate that physical inactivity and dietary patterns impact the onset of sarcopenia due to the decrease in muscle fiber size that begins at age 35 in sedentary individuals [10].

Another important factor for the onset of sarcopenia is the hormonal and inflammatory mechanisms present in chronic diseases and advanced age, leading to protein degradation [10].

3. Definition

EWGSOP2 defined sarcopenia as a progressive skeletal muscle disorder that impairs muscle function (quality) and mass (quantity) predisposing patients to a major likelihood of falls, fractures, physical disability, and mortality [5].

This new concept emphasizes the muscle function or quality, which is more important than the muscle quantity or mass parameter in the diagnosis of sarcopenia in the case of general population and CKD patients including those in hemodialysis [5].

This concept helps to identify and care for patients at risk of sarcopenia and establishes the basis for new and advanced definitions [5].

On the other hand, sarcopenia in the context of CKD is denominated as chronic kidney disease–related sarcopenia (CKD-RS) and includes hemodialysis and peritoneal dialysis patients. It is conceptualized as a progressive skeletal muscle disorder that impairs muscle function (quality) and mass (quantity) in the context of CKD and hemodialysis [3].

CKD is a syndrome characterized by uremic symptoms and alterations in the laboratory analyses due to abnormalities of kidney structure or/and function (estimated glomerular filtration rate < 60 ml/min/1.73 m2), present for a time > 3 months, according to the definition of KDIGO guidelines.

4. Pathophysiology

A healthy skeletal muscle depends on an adequate mechanism of degeneration, inflammation, regeneration, and remodeling-repair interrelated and time-dependent phases [11].

1. Degeneration phase: in this phase is secondary to necrosis of the skeletal muscle as a result of different injuries, a product of myofiber proteolysis for influx of intracellular calcium [11, 12].

2. Inflammatory phase: a product of myofiber necrosis, there is a high inflammatory response from both innate and adaptive immunities. Indeed, neutrophils, the first cell implicates, release free radicals and proteases, which generate the elimination of cellular debris and stimulate pro-inflammatory cytokines including homing macrophage cells (M1 and M2 types) [11, 12].

M1 macrophages, the abundant inflammatory cells, are responsible to produce pro-inflammatory cytokines, such as interleukin 12 (IL-12), tumor necrosis factor (TNF)-alpha, interleukin 1 (IL-1), and interleukin 6 (IL-6), and low amount of the anti-inflammatory interleukin 10 (IL-10). Indeed, they are capable of damaging host tissue [12].

M2 macrophages produce a high amount of anti-inflammatory interleukin 10 (IL-10), insulin-like growth factor-1 (IGF-1), and low pro-inflammatory interleukins, which can module the inflammatory responses, scavenge cellular debris, and promote angiogenesis and tissue remodeling and repair [12].

3. Regenerative phase: myoblasts constitute a pool of undifferentiated reserve muscle cells, and they are activated, proliferated, and then differentiated in skeletal muscle cells in response to the release at the injured site of growth factors, such as insulin-like growth factor-1 (IGF-1), hepatocyte growth factor (HGF), epidermal growth factor (EGF), transforming growth factors (TGF-a and TGF-b), and platelet-derived growth factors (PDGF-AA and PDGF-BB) [12].

Indeed, a high number of myoblast cells guarantee a major likelihood of mature skeletal muscle regeneration. Satellite cells play a principal role in this phase including muscle homeostasis [11, 12].

The mitotic capacity of the satellite cells has a limit and depends on the telomere shortening. As a result, during the proliferation phase, there is an inability to repair the muscle fiber [12].

4. Remodeling and repair phases: characterized by the regeneration of connective tissue, angiogenesis process, and function of skeletal muscle fibers that are damaged [11]. This is possible because of the formation of scar tissue, a product of the muscle injury, and the overproduction of all types of collagens secondary to the activation and overgrowth of extracellular matrix and transformation of growth factor-b1 (TGF-b1), which has been demonstrated to participate in the activation of the fibrosis cascade in the case of muscle injury [12].

Relationship of these phases to pathophysiology of CKD-RS is the association with a loss of skeletal muscle regeneration for a decreasing number of myoblasts, product of KDW characterized by a loss of body protein mass and fuel reserves in CKD and hemodialysis patients [11, 13].

This generates a lost of muscle mass, secondary to the following:

- High muscular fiber destruction (degeneration phase), product of a negative balance of protein homeostasis.

- Increased catabolism.

- Increment of pro-inflammatory cytokines (inflammatory phase) released by M1 macrophages.

- The direct association with the uremia syndrome, characterized by an imbalance in fluid/electrolytes, and acid-base homeostasis includes abnormal hormone function, a product of elevated serum urea and deterioration of the kidney filtrate [11, 13].

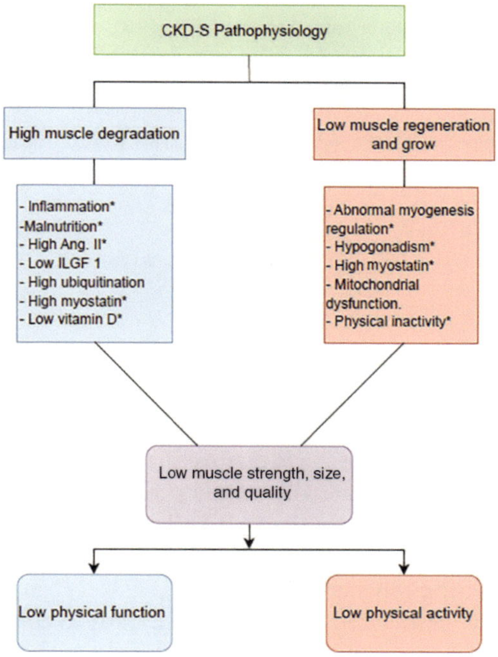

Figure 1.
Chronic kidney disease sarcopenia–related pathophysiology. Abbreviations: CKD-S: Chronic kidney disease sarcopenia related, Ang II: Angiotensin II; ILGF1: Insulin-like growth factor-1. Taken and modified to: Ref. [13].

Further in CKD-RS, an abnormal muscle regeneration phase (characteristic of normal aging) in early ages exists, secondary to a high activation of myostatin, a growth differentiation factor that is produced and released by myocytes of the skeletal muscle and acts on muscle cells to inhibit muscle growth and mass and that may be a pharmacologic target. Myostatin is inhibited to follistatin protein released by the liver in response to the exercise [13, 14].

In addition, hypogonadism is common in CKD and is associated with reduced muscle mass and strength and, thus, may be a target for skeletal muscle intervention in CKD [13]. Increased catabolism is attributed to different factors: uremic toxins, chronic inflammation, insulin resistance, hormonal imbalance, malnutrition, vitamin D deficiency, oxidative stress, and increased ubiquitination.

Vitamin D deficiency can upregulate the ubiquitin-proteasome (UPS) pathway leading to protein degradation and, subsequently, skeletal muscle atrophy [14].

The renin-angiotensin-aldosterone system is upregulated in CKD and impairs muscle regeneration and increases UPS proteolytic pathways. The UPS pathway degrades and digests ubiquitinated proteins through the activation of nuclear forkhead box members (FOXOs). In CKD, FOXO1 has been shown to play a role in CKD-related muscle wasting and could be a potential therapeutic target in future clinical studies. It is also important to note that patients with CKD often have comorbidities such as cardiomyopathy that also share pathways with sarcopenia such as oxidative stress and ghrelin, leptin, and cytokine release (**Figure 1**) [14].

Hemodialysis and CKD patients also are susceptible to KDW, a severe form of protein–energy wasting, secondary to the occurrence of PEW and cachexia, which increases the chance of sarcopenia [2].

Operational definition of sarcopenia in general population and CKD-RS
1. Probable sarcopenia: demonstrated by a decrease in muscle strength
2. Confirmed sarcopenia: low muscle quantity or quality demonstrated with additional assessment method
3. Severe sarcopenia: definitions 1 and 2 and very low physical performance demonstrated
Taken and modified to: Ref. [4].

Table 1.
Criteria for diagnosis of sarcopenia in CKD and hemodialysis patients [4].

5. Sarcopenia assessment and diagnosis

Sarcopenia in general population, CKD-RS, and hemodialysis patients is characterized by changes in a person's muscle quality that lead to a decreased muscle strength and muscle mass, which usually occurs at the beginning of the aging process or due to some chronic pathology, particularly inflammatory ones, such as CKD [15].

For this reason, diagnosis is given by measuring muscle strength and mass as the main parameter, as described in **Table 1**.

Various techniques to assess muscle quality are mostly available in clinical settings; physical performance was also considered part of the diagnosis but is now used to categorize the severity of sarcopenia.

EWGSOP proposed validated tools and tests for sarcopenia diagnosis in the general population without CKD and hemodialysis, which may be applied in hemodialysis patients because there is no consensus actually for this population [5].

Based on this, four criteria can be identified that must be recognized to diagnose sarcopenia in CKD-RS and hemodialysis patients [5]:

1. Screening of sarcopenia cases, through the use of the SARC-F questionnaire (low to moderate sensitivity and very high specificity) to predict a decreased muscle strength in ambulatory patients, or the Ishii score for the use at a hospital level [5].

2. Evaluate a case of positive screening sarcopenia, must be performed through the measurement of the decreased muscle strength in both the upper and lower limbs [5].

3. Confirm the sarcopenia diagnosis: there are several examinations with more complex and expensive devices that can be performed, such as bioelectrical impedance (BIA), dual-energy X-ray absorptiometry (DXA), magnetic resonance imaging, and muscle biopsy [5].

4. Finally, to determine the severity, physical performance tests related to locomotion are carried out, not only the muscles but also the nervous function and the balance part are assessed (**Table 2**) [5, 18].

6. Discussion

Sarcopenia syndrome is a muscular disease characterized by a loss of muscular mass and quality, resulting in low strength and function [3].

Evaluate	Measure tool	Research studies	Positive Cutoff points
To screen	SARC-F questionnaire Ishii screening tool Blood test	SARC-F Serum albumin	≥4 points < 3,5 mg/dl
To evaluate a case of positive case	Grip strength Chair stand test (chair rise test)	Grip strength Chair stand test (5 times sit-to-stand)	M: <27 kg W:<16 kg >15 s
To confirm diagnosis	Appendicular skeletal muscle mass (ASMM) by dual-energy X-ray absorptiometry (DXA) Whole-body skeletal muscle mass (SMM) or ASMM predicted by bioelectrical impedance analysis (BIA) Lumbar muscle cross-sectional area by CT or MRI	ASMM by DXA Whole-body SMM or ASMM by magnetic resonance imaging (MRI, total body protocol) Mid-thigh muscle cross-sectional area by computed tomography (CT) or MRI	M:<20 kg W:<15 kg
To determine severity	Gait speed Short physical performance battery (SPPB) Timed-up-and-go test (TUG) 400-meter walk or long-distance corridor walk (400-m walk)	Gait speed for 4.5 m (15 ft) SPPB TUG 400-m walk	Maximum duration Men: Height ≤ 173 cm ≥ 7 s Height > 173 cm ≥ 6 s Women: Height ≤ 159 cm ≥ 7 s Height > 159 cm ≥ 6 s ≤ 8 points ≥20 s Noncompletion or ≥ 6 min for completion
Anthropometric measurements to confirm diagnosis	Arm circumference Tricipital skin fold Arm muscle area	Prospective observational study Jiang. et al. [16]	[17] Men < 26.3 cm Women <25.2 cm Men >65 years old <6 mm Women >65 years old < 14 mm Men < 24.5 cm Women <19.6 cm

Abbreviations: M: men; W: women; Kg: kilograms; s seconds. m: meters.
Taken and modificated to: Ref. [4].

Table 2.
Screening and diagnosis assessment for chronic kidney disease–related sarcopenia [4, 5].

We recommend the concept of CKD-RS to mention a CKD patient undergoing renal replacement treatment (hemodialysis or peritoneal dialysis) with a diagnosis of sarcopenia.

Sarcopenia has a prevalence between 10 and 27% in older age population without renal kidney disease (> 60 age); however, in CKD and renal replacement treatment patients, the prevalence is higher (28.5–40.3%) and is associated with poor outcomes [8].

With the high prevalence of frailty in this population, other syndromes inter-related with sarcopenia increase the possibility of high mortality and poor outcomes too. A prospective observational study determined a prevalence of 67.5 % of frailty in patients at the beginning of dialysis [18].

This high prevalence in older ages and in CKD patients independent of age is due to a high muscular fiber destruction for a negative balance of protein homeostasis with an increased catabolism, inadequate mechanism of degeneration, inflammation, regeneration, and remodeling-repair phases on the skeletal muscle [10, 14].

Another important cause in aging patients is the muscular alterations related with the senescence (shorting telomere present on the satellite muscular cells and regenerative skeletal muscle function) with abnormal neuromuscular integrity and muscle fat content, a product of an alteration in the homeostasis of the endocrine system, sex hormones, inadequate nutrition, malabsorption, muscle disuse, and concomitant diseases and cachexia [4, 12].

The most important mechanism of sarcopenia in CKD is the uremia syndrome responsible for a negative balance of protein homeostasis, followed by an abnormal muscle regeneration phase (characteristic of normal aging) in early ages, secondary to a high activation of myostatin (protein responsible to inhibit the skeletal muscle growth) [13].

Increased catabolism is the most important mechanism in renal replacement treatment patients attributed to different factors, such as uremic toxins, chronic inflammation, insulin resistance, hormonal imbalance, malnutrition, vitamin D deficiency, and oxidative stress [14].

Hemodialysis and peritoneal dialysis patients also are susceptible to KDW, a severe form of protein-energy wasting, that aggregates more risk of sarcopenia and finally cachexia [2].

Thus, CKD patients are more susceptible to sarcopenia syndrome independent of the age, secondary to a lot of intrinsic (previously reviewed) and extrinsic factors.

Extrinsic factors are added to the intrinsic factor, such as comorbidities: hypertension, diabetes, cardiac diseases, inflammatory diseases, infections, and immunosuppression. In patients on renal replacement therapy, is add the extracorporeal treatment and the vascular access (catheter dialysis, peritoneal catheter or arteria-venous fistula), that predispose to a major probability of infections, hypercatabolic and hyperinflammatory state.

Currently, scales used for sarcopenia screening and diagnosis are the SARC-F score and the modified SARC-assisted CalF score, reviewed in a meta-analysis that discovered a sensitivity of SARC-F low to moderate (28.9–55.3%) and so was its specificity (68.9–88.9%). Although SARC-CalF is associated with higher specificity (87.7–91.3%), its sensitivity is not satisfactory (45.9–57.2%) [19].

Furthermore, a lot of studies have developed a risk prediction nomogram for sarcopenia in hemodialysis patients, based on different parameters such as C-reactive protein, body mass index, mid-upper arm muscle circumference, old age (> 60), serum phosphorus (< 1.13 mmol/L), low body mass index (< 18.5 kg/m^2), calf circumference, and serum creatinine [19].

However, these nomograms need more studies to validate and guarantee a better sensibility and specificity for the diagnosis of CKD-RS. At the same time, other scales such as SARC-F and SARC-assisted CalF score need more studies to consider application in the general population including CKD and hemodialysis patients.

Exist other scales with good validation such as The Asian Working Group for Sarcopenia (AWGS) 2019, used in a lot of investigation studies for development nomograms for sarcopenia in hemodialysis patients, that we consider is not applicable to our population because the variation of body mass index and muscle mass parameters.

Consequently, we recommend for the diagnostic of CKD-RS patients undergoing hemodialysis and without the methods proposed by The European Working Group on Sarcopenia in Older People (EWGSOP), which despite being validated in the general population without CKD and hemodialysis, may be able to applicate in these patients because for the time there's not a consensus for this population [5].

Thus, the following steps are necessary for a proper diagnosis: first screening sarcopenia (SARC-F questionnaire in ambulatory patients or the Ishii score for hospitalized patients), evaluating a case of positive screening sarcopenia (measurement of the decreased muscle strength in upper and lower limbs), confirming sarcopenia diagnosis BIA, DXA, magnetic resonance imaging, and muscle biopsy), and determining the severity (physical performance tests) [5, 20].

In the majority of cases, it is not possible to confirm CKD-RS with BIA, DXA, magnetic resonance imaging, or muscle biopsy, because it is either expensive or not available. However, the screening and confirmation with measurement of the decreased muscle strength for the distinct methods are sufficient to confirm the diagnosis.

Finally, the diagnosis of sarcopenia through a precise diagnostic test, applicable for CKD and renal replacement treatment patients, is primordial, due to the high prevalence in this population group and the high susceptibility to other comorbidities.

More validation studies related to the diagnosis of CKD-RS scores are necessary. Therefore, the implementation of other clinical diagnostic criteria such as serum albumin and anthropometric measurements such as arm circumference and tricipital skinfold should be considered, which could be useful in these cases.

Author details

Santiago David Silva Tobar[1*] and Leticia Andreina Lozada Tobar[2]

1 Nephrologist, Department of Nephrology, General Docente Ambato Hospital and SOLCA Núcleo Tungurahua Hospital, Ambato, Ecuador

2 Nutrition and Dietetics Universidad Técnica de Ambato, Ecuador

*Address all correspondence to: sdst1986@gmail.com

References

[1] Eknoyan G, Lameire N, UweEckardt K, et al. KDIGO 2012 clinical practice guideline for the evaluation and management of chronic kidney disease. Journal of the International Society of Nephrology 2013;**3**(1):5-14. Available from: http://www.kidney-international.org

[2] Fouque D, Kalantar-Zadeh K, Kopple J, et al. A proposed nomenclature and diagnostic criteria for protein-energy wasting in acute and chronic kidney disease. Kidney International. 2008;**73**(4):391-398. DOI: 10.1038/sj.ki.5002585. Epub 2007 Dec 19. Erratum in: Kidney Int. 2008 Aug;74(3):393. Trevinho-Becerra, A (corrected to Treviño-Becerra, A)

[3] Elder M, Moonen A, Crowther S, et al. Chronic kidney disease-related sarcopenia as a prognostic indicator in elderly haemodialysis patients. BMC Nephrology. 2023;**24**:138. DOI: 10.1186/s12882-023-03175-5

[4] Cruz-Jentoft AJ, Baeyens JP, Bauer JM, et al. Sarcopenia: European consensus on definition and diagnosis: Report of the European working group on sarcopenia in older people. Sarcopenia: European consensus on definition and diagnosis: Report of the European working group on sarcopenia in older people. Age and Ageing. 2010;**39**(4):412-423. DOI: 10.1093/ageing/afq034

[5] Cruz-Jentoft AJ, Bahat G, Bauer J, et al. Writing Group for the European Working Group on sarcopenia in older people 2 (EWGSOP2), and the extended group for EWGSOP2. Sarcopenia: Revised European consensus on definition and diagnosis. Age and Ageing. 2019;**48**(1):16-31. DOI: 10.1093/ageing/afy169. Erratum in: Age Ageing. 2019;48(4):601

[6] Petermann-Rocha F, Balntzi V, Gray SR, Lara J, Ho FK, Pell JP, et al. Global prevalence of sarcopenia and severe sarcopenia: A systematic review and meta-analysis. Journal of Cachexia, Sarcopenia and Muscle. 2022;**13**(1):86-99. DOI: 10.1002/jcsm.12783. Epub 2021 Nov 23

[7] Shafiee G, Keshtkar A, Soltani A, Ahadi Z, Larijani B, Heshmat R. Prevalence of sarcopenia in the world: A systematic review and meta-analysis of general population studies. Journal of Diabetes and Metabolic Disorders. 2017;**16**:21. DOI: 10.1186/s40200-017-0302-x

[8] Fu C, Yan D, Wang L, Duan F, Gu D, Yao N, et al. High prevalence of sarcopenia and myosteatosis in patients undergoing hemodialysis. Frontiers in Endocrinology (Lausanne) [Internet]. 2023;**14**:7-9. DOI: 10.3389/fendo.2023.1117438

[9] Yuan S, Larsson SC. Epidemiology of sarcopenia: Prevalence, risk factors, and consequences. Metabolism. 2023;**144**:155533. DOI: 10.1016/j.metabol.2023.155533. Epub 2023 Mar 11

[10] Barberi L, Scicchitano BM, De Rossi M, Bigot A, Duguez S, Wielgosik A, et al. Age-dependent alteration in muscle regeneration: The critical role of tissue niche. Biogerontology. 2013;**14**(3):273-292. DOI: 10.1007/s10522-013-9429-4. Epub 2013 May 12

[11] Carosio S, Berardinelli MG, Aucello M, Musarò A. Impact of ageing on muscle cell regeneration. Ageing

Research Reviews. 2011;**10**(1):35-42. DOI: 10.1016/j.arr.2009.08.001. Epub 2009 Aug 13

[12] Fahal IH. Uraemic sarcopenia: Aetiology and implications. Nephrology, Dialysis, Transplantation. 2014;**29**(9):1655-1665. DOI: 10.1093/ndt/gft070. Epub 2013 Apr 25

[13] Moorthi RN, Avin KG. Clinical relevance of sarcopenia in chronic kidney disease. Current Opinion in Nephrology and Hypertension. 2017;**26**(3):219-228. DOI: 10.1097/MNH.0000000000000318

[14] Erdogan T, Catikkas NM, Oren MM, et al. Ishii test for screening sarcopenia: Performance in community-dwelling older adults. Aging Clinical and Experimental Research. 2022;**34**(4):785-791. DOI: 10.1007/s40520-021-01998-6. Epub 2021 Oct 15

[15] Sánchez-Tocino ML, Miranda-Serrano B, Gracia-Iguacel C, de -Alba-Peñaranda AM, Mas-Fontao S, López-González A, et al. Sarcopenia assessed by 4-step EWGSOP2 in elderly hemodialysis patients: Feasibility and limitations. PLoS One [Internet]. 2022;**17**(1):e0261459. DOI: 10.1371/journal.pone.0261459

[16] Jiang K, Slee A, Davemport A. American Society for Parenteral and Enteral Nutrition. September. 2020;**30**. DOI: 10.1002/ncp.10597

[17] Lee RC, Wang Z, Heo M, Ross R, Janssen I, Heymsfield SB. Total-body skeletal muscle mass: development and cross-validation of anthropometric prediction models. The American Journal of Clinical Nutrition. 2000;**72**(3):796-803. DOI: 10.1093/ajcn/72.3.796

[18] Silva S, Milano C, García G, et al. Frailty at the beginning of dialysis; is it a prognostic factor ? Journal of Renal Endocrinology. 2021;7:4-6. DOI: 10.34172/jre.2021.13. Available from: http://www.jrenendo.com

[19] Cai G, Ying J, Pan M, Lang X, Yu W, Zhang Q. Development of a risk prediction nomogram for sarcopenia in hemodialysis patients. BMC Nephrology. 2022;**23**(1):319. DOI: 10.1186/s12882-022-02942-0

[20] Voelker SN, Michalopoulos N, Maier AB, Reijnierse EM. Reliability and concurrent validity of the SARC-F and its modified versions: A systematic review and meta-analysis. Journal of the American Medical Directors Association. 2021;**22**(9):1864-1876.e16. DOI: 10.1016/j.jamda.2021.05.011

Chapter 4

Perspective Chapter: The Strategy of Motivation Technique in Sarcopenia Prevention

Katdel Istifanus Dafup

Abstract

Because of the difficulties in sarcopenia management caused by the scarce pharmacologic agents for cure, and the influence of lifestyle in rendering the disease course reversible, prevention of sarcopenia becomes a primary care need. The interventions prone to reducing the development of sarcopenia are non-pharmacological, mainly requiring lifestyle modification—a primary care intervention. The sarcopenic elderly require self-motivation to sustain their independence in lifestyle practice, as many struggle with apathy; without motivation, they may relapse even after attaining cure. Hence, "Motivational Interviewing (MI)" is an emerging promising behavioural technique for sarcopenic elderly to initiate and maintain a positive lifestyle. Primary care physicians play a role in identifying those at risk and initiating this behavioural technique as a prevention strategy; also, by making early diagnosis, the primary care physician refers the sarcopenic for specialist care and classifies those with comorbidities or severity for coordination of a comprehensive care.

Keywords: sarcopenia, motivational interviewing, lifestyle changes, primary care, prevention, motivation, patient, therapist

1. Introduction

The prevention of sarcopenia is a need in primary care [1, 2]. This is important so because Primary Care, as reported by the WHO in 2021, is the healthcare space that offers the initial care of patients in a coordinated, continuous, comprehensive and patient-centric manner. This makes primary care a significant domain in health promotion and disease prevention—including the prevention of sarcopenia [3]. Due to the several undesirable effects ascribed to sarcopenia on the elderly, and the difficulties in its management in general, this chapter highlights the merits of sarcopenia prevention and introduces the concept of a behavioural technique in prevention; while buttressing the primary care setting as a suitable care point for this task [4].

Preventing sarcopenia becomes necessary in primary care, firstly because there are hardly any pharmacologic agents for cure [1, 5]. As of now, the prime treatment for sarcopenia is non-pharmacotherapy. However, there are prospects of reliable and sustainable outcomes with pharmacotherapy for the sarcopenic elderly [6]. "*Clinical trials of new drugs targeting multiple molecules are ongoing*" [6]. Pharmacotherapy is

 IntechOpen

the use of drugs to effect clinical improvement in the course of sarcopenia or positively modify its progression [6]; while non-pharmacological treatment entails the use of other forms of treatment not requiring the use of drugs or medicine [6, 7]. In sarcopenia management, non-pharmacologic prevention and treatment have been based on lifestyle modification and the use of dietary supplements [6]. These lifestyle measures for reducing the onset or progression of sarcopenia are mostly physical exercise and dietary control. Those measures are interventions in primary care, often requiring the role of primary care physicians [1, 8]. Primary care is the initial medical attention at the potential, or earlier onset, or progression of the disease [9]. Thus, lifestyle measures confer great benefits in sarcopenia care, whether in the prevention or treatment of its severity [1, 5]. Lifestyle is termed as the deliberate practice of a routine that affects the long-term social course of a habit or behavioural pattern, like substance, alcohol or tobacco use, dietary habits, and physical activity and sedentariness, thereby impacting the overall health of people [1]. "*Physical activity is defined as any movement produced by the contraction of skeletal muscles causing increases in energy expenditure*" while "*sedentary behavior refers to activities that do not substantially increase energy expenditure above the resting level*" [5]. Various researchers have suggested the effects of lifestyle modification on distinct measures of sarcopenia like muscle mass or strength and physical performance [1, 5, 8, 10, 11].

Secondly, primary care is at the heart of sarcopenia prevention because the prevention can be effective with the primary care physician due to his/her acquaintance with the health behaviour pattern among patients, performing a significant role in prevention [1, 2]. Furthermore, the need for the primary care provider's acquaintance is because the disease course, being influenced by lifestyle, is reversible [1, 2, 12].

In the early onset of sarcopenia development known as the pre-sarcopenia, there is the manifestation of a reduction in skeletal muscle build of the affected elderly [10]. If not managed, pre-sarcopenia may cause the development of sarcopenia, leading to a high risk of geriatric frailty and falls [10]. There is a disturbing experiential connection between geriatric frailty and sarcopenia. This fragility is known to cause debility and loss of self-abilities with an increased risk of geriatric untimely deaths. These conditions can all be averted if pre-sarcopenia is tackled by preventing the manifestation of sarcopenia features to forestall lingering bodily deterioration [10]. However, after a cure, patients with sarcopenic presentations who get treated may revert to their old pre-sarcopenic state [3]. This could happen because when one does not have self-motivation for personal improvement, the individual is mostly highly physically inactive, committed to unhealthy diets, consuming alcohol and, or using tobacco. That individual, for instance, may not indulge in frequent social events, partake in recreational activities which increase physical activity and harbour innumerable health benefits [3]. The effect of ageing on mental health has been strongly suggested to have a relationship with the apathy the geriatric display towards lifestyle change which is a necessity in the prevention and treatment of sarcopenia [3]. Some of the reasons for the ambivalence to lifestyle modification in the elderly stem from: loneliness and hopelessness leading to social isolation; loss of independence leading to the feeling loss of self-identity; physical symptoms relating to chronic pain leading to physical and emotional exhaustion; neurological changes leading to cognitive decline; the fear of the overall ageing process leading to anxiety about death and dying; and, loss of loved ones leading to worsening loneliness, depression and being somnolent [3].

Consequently, an approach to counselling linking improvement or maintenance of physical well-being to behaviour change called "Motivational Interviewing (MI)" has been studied and strongly suggested to be beneficial for patients to recover "self-efficacy" for lifestyle change [1, 3]. Hence, a sarcopenic individual requires self-motivation to address ambivalence and sustain independence in lifestyle practice which would advance the quality of prevention [3, 9]. Many geriatrics struggle with apathy or a loss of motivation [3, 13]. Without self-motivation, even those who attain a cure may relapse [3]. Many health-based studies have proposed the merits of MI in the prevention and treatment of several enduring health conditions, and those requiring lifestyle change among the elderly [13, 14]. By that implication, many senior citizens who need to make dire lifestyle changes to manage their prevailing chronic medical conditions would require MI. Hence with MI, the elderly can imbibe lifestyle modifications much genuinely easier by using MI as a means for attaining and sustaining self-efficacy [2].

This chapter seeks to highlight the role of the primary care physician in the management of sarcopenia; and point to the benefits of MI—behavioural counselling technique in primary care management of chronic diseases that could be adopted, with benefits, as a primary care technique in sarcopenia prevention and treatment strategy for assisting especially, the susceptible elderly.

2. Prevention of sarcopenia is better than cure

The prevalence of sarcopenia is of epidemiologic proportion owing to its relatedness with exposure to specific risk factors [5]. Senility is reportedly a major risk from ageing dynamics relating to physiological changes affecting the human body systems [1, 5, 8]. From late youthful age to the onset of elderly age, there is a projected yearly gain of roughly 0.45 kg (1 lb) of fat and shedding of about 0.23 kg (0.5 lb) of muscle [5]. Also, from the onset of ageing, there is an estimated yearly loss of 2% of muscle bulk with a concomitant annual loss of muscle strength of about 3% [5]. The consequences of these losses are a reduction in muscle bulk together with deposition of fat tissue triggering a physique configuration known as "*sarcopenic obesity which is related to changes in skeletal muscle tissue and low muscle quality disarrangements of myofilaments, accumulation of reactive oxidative species, and reduction in satellite cell activity and number*" [5]. Hence, sarcopenia prevalence is reportedly high among the elderly and increases with age [1, 2, 5], possibly reaching a proportion as high as 1 in 2 by age 80 years [5], with a higher male-to-female ratio [1–3]. Furthermore, as the universal life expectancy rises, the frequency of geriatrics in human populations seems to be on the rise, the world over [5]. Therefore, the frequency of sarcopenia is also potentially on a surge [5]. Similarly, there is a potential increase in its burden on requirements for human, financial and health resources [5, 11]. The financial burden, for example, can be regarded from various unswerving facts like the bills of medical care of a sarcopenic; while secondarily, the economic burden arises from the sarcopenic being unproductive [5]. Yet, at present, there is no cure for sarcopenia [8, 15]. Consequently, developing strategies to prevent sarcopenia continues to be of greater importance, and a potentially more rewarding approach than focusing on its cure [5, 15]. This aligns with the common axiom in public health practice that "*prevention is better than cure*". This suggests that disease deterrence is fundamental in the future of individuals, including the elderly healthy living. Thus, it portends a lot of sense to deter the occurrence of sarcopenia rather than to suffer the menace it inflicts on the individual, family, and society.

Aside from the above mentioned, ageing—a notable non-modifiable risk factor of sarcopenia, there are modifiable lifestyle conditions like physical inactivity, inadequate nutrition, cigarette smoking, and alcohol consumption, implicated in the development of sarcopenia [1, 5]. The existence of lifestyle factors in its aetiology, with scarce drugs for its treatment, suggests the merit of primary care intervention for prevention of the condition... Also, in order to prevent complications of chronic diseases like sarcopenia, lifestyle intervention has been reported as a necessity [2]. The subsequent discussion highlights how modification of those lifestyle factors could impact the outlook of sarcopenia management in primary care.

An important lifestyle factor of sarcopenia prevention in primary practice includes "physical activity" which comprises of "*intentional movements for health benefits such as brisk walk or biking, as well as daily activities such as standing up from a chair and climbing stairs*". Thus, when individuals execute solely routine physical activities like to stand and walk slowly, or lift light items, they are tagged "*inactive*". However, the primary care physician could advise the addition of "*intentional movements*" to the routine physical activities to yield improved well-being for the sarcopenic elderly. Another way to improve physical activity is by "*exercise*" which is an intentional movement that is "*intentionally fashioned in a recurring physical motion executed at will for the maintenance or improvement of bodily fitness, functioning, and wellbeing*" [5]. The lifestyle of physical activity guarantees that the elderly gains increased muscle mass and strength, and becomes less prone to the onset of sarcopenia [5]. Another activity-related lifestyle factor to sarcopenia development is sedentariness, which refers to a behaviour of doing bodily movements of about equal level of energy expenditure as the resting level activities like sleeping, sitting, lying down, and watching television [5]. Sedentariness is an implicated factor in the development of life-long illnesses, frailty, as well sarcopenia. Thus, in the elderly, being immobile favours loss of muscle bulk especially in the distal extremities by interrupting protein metabolism, favouring the catabolic rather than the anabolic process of skeletal muscle protein synthesis [5]. This is just as reported by a study in which immobilised animals showed skeletal muscle damage in old animals compared to young ones in relation to activation of several proteolytic systems which were activated in the animals' muscles following inactivity [3].

Since reduced body movement and sedentariness are core factors of sarcopenia manifestation, physical activity and exercise are strategies in primary care for the prevention and treatment of sarcopenia [3]. For this, resistance exercise alone, or with aerobics, can be used to improve the muscle volume and strength in the elderly [3]. Aerobic exercise is one that "*involves continued bulky muscles movement contributing less to muscle hypertrophy but increasing the thickness of the muscle fibers, and biomolecular activities*" [3]. Through these "cardio" exercises like jogging, skipping, and brisk walking, there is a reduction of age-related damages in muscle catabolism which influences the insulin and mammalian target of rapamycin (mTOR) signalling pathways to induce a reduction in skeletal muscle adipose tissue, thereby causing improvement in muscle activity [3]. Thus, "*aerobic training in older adults improves nutrient delivery to muscles, thereby inducing an increased anabolic effect of nutrient intake*". On the other hand, resistance exercise, which is "*a form of exercise in which muscle contraction occurs against an external load*", displays a far-reaching result with regards to building muscle bulk and strength and reduces the progression of sarcopenia [3]. Examples of resistance training include heavy weight lifting, sprinting, and push-ups, which work by increasing muscle bulk by directly triggering muscle protein synthesis within just a few hours of a brief session of workout [3]. "*During resistance workouts, enzymatic activation of mTOR leads to activation of extracellular signal-regulated kinases 1/2 (ERK1/2) and mitogen-activated protein kinase (MAPK) leading to downstream translation of factors prompting muscle protein formation*" [3]. Overall, the success of resistance exercise stems from improvement in muscle bulk and strength in the sarcopenic geriatric. Additionally, an increase in muscle strength in older adults is reportedly achieved with as little as one resistance training session per week, similar to the way a resistance exercise would in a 3-day per week programme [3].

Inadequate intake from diverse factors relating to both physiologic and socioeconomic realms in the elderly results in poor nutrition, which is another important risk factor in the development of sarcopenia [3]. Protein intake by the elderly is related to the mechanisms underlying sarcopenia via its influence on the skeletal muscle metabolism. The recommended dietary allowance (RDA) of protein is 0.8 g/kg/day, with greater requirements in geriatrics (1.14 g/kg/day) compared to the youths (0.8 g/kg/day); yet, nearly half of seniors over 70 years fall short of the recommendation [3]. The high protein requirements in geriatrics are likely due to the phenomenon of "*anabolic resistance*",—"*a blunted response of muscle protein synthesis in the elderly relative to the young following ingestion of dietary protein*". Also, Leucine, an amino acid contained in some proteins, is vital in controlling muscle protein metabolic process by the translational control leading to activation of the mTOR signalling pathway and it is known as an "*anti-atrophic agent*" [2, 3]. The toxic level of leucine supplementation is uncommon therefore, supplementing it for the elderly is a possible future primary care strategy to prevent the development of sarcopenia [3]. Meanwhile, primary care nutritional education/advice for the elderly should be towards consumption of essential amino acids (EAAs) rich diets particularly leucine-rich dietary sources like beef, fish, and legumes [3]. The recommended least level, 1.2 g, of proteins/kg/day for the elderly could be augmented if there is catabolism or muscle loss. Aside from protein, there is also the information that vitamin D serves an imperative function in skeletal muscle tissue which preserves the integrity of type II fibres, thereby conserving bodily strength and preventing falls. The elderly are prone to vitamin D deficiency because their skin and kidneys lose the efficient ability for production and conversion, respectively, of vitamin D. Hence, supplementing vitamin D in the elderly is another potentially key approach, in preventing and treating sarcopenia in primary care [3]. The primary care provider has the responsibility to advise dietary or nutritional supplementation, or offer supplemental vitamin D pills to the required elderly; this should be combined with exercise intervention sarcopenia management [2].

Although alcohol consumption is believed to play a role in the development of sarcopenia, the pathway is purportedly indirectly by promoting loss of muscle bulk and strength in the elderly [3]. Thus, chronic alcohol consumption is a negative behaviour that recurrently causes features of low muscle mass and strength, muscle pain, cramps, difficulties in gait, and falls, and ultimately favouring onset of sarcopenia [3]. "*This phenomenon is known as alcoholic myopathy*" [3]. Acute form of the myopathy could rarely manifest following binge drinking in undernourished alcoholics presenting with muscle aches and wasting with the concomitant urinary loss of myoglobin leading to impaired renal function. Conversely, a commoner myopathy manifesting in about half of all chronic alcoholics is characterised by nutritional deficiencies and, or alcoholic hepatitis which could be ameliorated through abstinence within about a year. "*This chronic alcoholic myopathy causes wasting of about 30% of muscle mass through programmed atrophy of type II muscle fibers*" [3]. Therefore, counselling on reducing alcohol consumption may be a worthy primary care strategy for the prevention of sarcopenia [3].

Cigarette smoking is another lifestyle factor implicated in the development of sarcopenia as it relates to negative health habits like physical inactivity and nutritional deficiencies [3]. Smoking is reported to fairly lessen appendicular skeletal muscle mass, and smokers with sarcopenia tend to smoke significantly more. Overall, tobacco smoking is a risk factor for sarcopenia and tobacco cessation counselling is an important sarcopenia prevention in the primary care setting [3].

Overall, behaviours relating to diet, exercise, consumption of alcohol and tobacco have significant bearing on the development of sarcopenia in the elderly, and its prevention and treatment. In order to delay the onset of sarcopenia or treat it, the choices of lifestyle must be considered seriously. While physiological and systemic bodily changes that ensue during ageing and accelerate the development of sarcopenia are not easily controllable, lifestyle factors are far more modifiable. Therefore, health education and counselling on lifestyle with regards to prevention of the development of sarcopenia in the elderly is of great importance in primary care management of the disorder [3, 15]. Since sarcopenia worsens the geriatrics' quality of life in physical, functional, emotional, cognitive, and economic domains, to mention the least, preventive strategies in terms of primary care have been strongly recommended by some research and health organisations like the European Working Group on Sarcopenia in Older People (EWGSOP) [3] and European Society for Clinical and Economic Aspects of Osteoporosis and Osteoarthritis (ESCEO) [8]. Also, AWGS in 2019 recommended that individuals diagnosed with "possible sarcopenia", should start lifestyle interventions and receive related health education from primary healthcare providers [2]. The primary care provider is also encouraged to formulate institutionalised guidelines for sarcopenia screening and assessment tools as a preventive strategy since screening assists early detection of individuals at risk of sarcopenia [16].

3. Prevention of sarcopenia: the primary care need

The primary care setting helps as the foremost service area for patients. It is a vital point where health promotion and disease prevention can be offered. This, therefore, underscores the necessity of sarcopenia care in the primary care setting which also represents the foremost location for continuous, comprehensive, and coordinated care that is individualistic and undifferentiated. Hence, the constraint of the first contact clinician to deal with a barrage of elderly problems risks sarcopenia development. This challenge is however surmounted in primary care, by the development of several tools of varying sensitivity and specificity that assist in the assessment and preventive therapies of sarcopenia. Typically, referral to a higher level of care may be required because a good assessment has been made in primary care [1].

The diagnosis of sarcopenia is a great task in primary care and some higher settings, classically because of the practice of requiring magnetic resonance imaging (MRI) and computed tomography (CT) scans for the non-invasive diagnosis. This poses a limitation in primary care practice due to the difficulty in availability, affordability, and expert manpower requirements for the use of such gadgets. Consequent to the aforementioned challenges which also bedevil higher levels of care, anthropometry in primary care settings has been suggested as a worthwhile tool. This assists primary care physicians in recognising patients at risk of sarcopenia and identifying the need for collaborative care [1–8]. Not making an early diagnosis is a major impediment to the treatment of sarcopenia and it also deters the prospect of preventive intervention. Similarly, there is evidence suggesting that there is no particular biomarker specifically for sarcopenia diagnosis. However, only a combination of numerous biomarkers is suggested to help accurate diagnosis; and a good primary care practice curtails this problem. The EWGSOP diagnostic criterion provides a detailed diagnostic process; however, it is multistep, time-consuming, and costly [10]. To curb this challenge of diagnostic intricacy in primary care, Beaudart et al. proffered a diagnostic context that is practicable and could be adopted in primary care [12]. Based on that guideline, sarcopenia can be diagnosed in primary care based on: (a) best recommended tool which involves: speed gait and handgrip strength; or (b) best alternative tool which involves: anthropometric measurements and repeated chair stand test; or (c) less recommended tool which involves: DXA, CT-scan, MRI, BIA, lower limb muscle strength, timed up-and-go test, balance test, 6-minute walk test, 400 m walk test, stair climb test and Short Physical Performance Battery (SPPB) [8]. It is reported summarily, that: "*the prime assessment of muscle bulk is by DXA, which if not accessible, some anthropometric parameters could be simply measured in the first contact care settings as important initial screening of those elderly with reduced muscle bulk. These patients should further be referred for advanced evaluation by the required specialist*" [8].

With respect to the contemporary challenges in consensus regarding unremarkable concerns relating to the limitation of time and availability of assessment tools for sarcopenia diagnosis in the primary care settings, the role of primary care physicians would be to offer assessment of risk for sarcopenia, undertake early diagnosis of sarcopenia, and to refer them to the specialists for treatment [8]. A new perspective now is the requirement for the family physician to offer behaviour change education and advice, and counselling intervention for prevention of sarcopenia in those at risk [17]. For this, it has been found that some evidence abounds about the success of motivational approaches in management of the elderly with such chronic disease conditions as sarcopenia. However, studies applying motivational strategies for sarcopenic elderly are scarce [17].

Furthermore, "secondary care" in sarcopenia management still depends on adherence to lifestyle change as well as modification of its comorbid risks like hypertension, hypercholesterolemia, diabetes, and obesity [1, 5, 12, 18]. These comorbid conditions are non-communicable conditions also related to lifestyle that may co-exist with sarcopenia [1]. They are very common in primary care settings, and lifestyle modification endeavours can likewise support their management just as sarcopenia management by providing additional treatment benefits [3, 19]. The role of the primary care provider here is to assist the sarcopenic to have comprehensive care by coordinating the requirement for an interdisciplinary management in this case [1].

4. Motivation technique, a primary care prevention of sarcopenia

Although people change their personalities slightly as they get older, this is different from the deliberate behavioural change required in lifestyle modification for disease prevention [18, 19]. A personality is the constitutional tendency of an individual to display a set of habits while behaviour is an acquired set of habits based on repetitive actions that have been mastered over time [20]. The behavioural technique is a process of mentally analysing behaviour patterns, permitting individuals to discover their personalities and individual values [9, 10]. This has been used in clinical practice to evoke behavioural change that is necessary for disease prevention [18, 19]. Patients are made to discover and value what means the most to them at each stage of change [2]. Motivational techniques assist the potential sarcopenic to make behavioural changes by aiming, targeting, and getting committed to a changed lifestyle which prevents the course of the disease and tolerably reduces the healthcare cost.

Largely, through motivation for change, the sarcopenic elderly begin a regular positive lifestyle [9]. To develop strategies to prevent and treat sarcopenia, the risk factors and causes of sarcopenia must be identified [10, 12]. Some of these risks are routine behaviours having a major impact on health and the onset of sarcopenia [10, 11]. The development of sarcopenia is also impacted by the complex changes of ageing related to lifestyle habits [10]. These habits include impaired nutrition, sedentariness, alcohol and tobacco use. These lifestyle factors have been reported to harm skeletal muscle strength and the development of sarcopenia [9, 10].

A common motivational technique used in primary care is "Motivational Interviewing" [13, 14]. "*It is a behaviour change technique that has a specific focus on increasing confidence*", and solving the patient's ambivalence in a collaborative way in order to increase physical activity in chronic diseases like sarcopenia [13, 14]. There has been a growing body of evidence about motivational interviewing ability to cause health behaviour change in chronic medical conditions [14]. Also, evidence abounds about the reliability of the technique in leading to a remarkable rise in physical activity among people with chronic health conditions [14].

The knowledge of the modifiable behavioural factors makes primary care a top point of care for sarcopenia. At this level, patient education, with discussions tailored to attract the patient's consideration to the calamitous problems of sarcopenia like loss of muscle strength, ease of trauma, frequent hospital admissions, and loss of activities of daily living [8, 9]. This education process necessitates an advanced level of enduring self-determination from the patient called motivation to change. Motivational interviewing is the crucial step for success in motivating the individual for health behaviour change [8, 21]. Being an evidence-based behavioural therapy, Motivational Interviewing (MI) is proposed for supporting health behaviour change [21]. MI was initially useful in supporting behaviour change in the treatment of substance dependency and alcoholism, but it has currently gained evidence of usefulness in the prevention and treatment of chronic disorders like obesity and type 2 diabetes mellitus; and now, it is presenting a promise of success in sarcopenia care by being effective in promoting behavioural change [21].

Physical activity as a behaviour is viewed as a set of planned actions like exercises at home or in the clinic, with the target of sarcopenia prevention by preventing muscle weakness or loss of bulk [9]. There have been reports from research strongly linking social components to behaviour change among geriatrics to enhance their enthusiasm [9]. For instance, organising group fitness programmes for the elderly or daily home-workout with family members are good approaches because many elderly relish physical exercises [9]. However, despite these tactics to improve participation in exercise activities, without the motivational technique—which pursues improvement in individual's self-efficacy and motivation, physical activity would not be sufficiently initiated or maintained. On the other hand, participation in exercise activity would lead to remarkable preventive health outcomes [9].

Although there is a paucity of research on motivational techniques in the care of sarcopenia, evidence however abounds on the potential success of motivational approaches among the elderly with several lifestyle disorders. There exist other approaches to "motivate and empower" geriatrics to prevent the onset of frailty and sarcopenia by behavioural modification [13]. The motivation of the elderly can be performed using established behavioural models: cognitive-behavioural therapy, the health belief model, and motivational interviewing [13]. "*Cognitive-behavioural therapy is a directive approach to increase motivation by eliminating the negative thoughts that hinder functioning. This is because in the sarcopenic elderly, the mood of self-incompetence can restrict execution of workouts, predominantly in elderly with comorbid conditions and/or low physical/functional levels*" [13]. Although cognitive-behavioural interventions have equally been suggested to express effectiveness in increasing physical activity also in older adults, the therapy focuses on changing undesirable thought patterns and behaviours. Whereas in motivational interviewing, a non-directive but more collaborative strategy is used to prompt a discussion about, as well as address, the patient's ambivalence [13]. Another behavioural model used to motivate people to participate in exercise as a treatment for diabetes and frailty is the health belief model (HBM). HBM has been widely applied to other areas of health behaviours [13]. Of all these behavioural approaches, motivational interviewing is gaining usefulness in clinical practice because of its proven success in the prevention and treatment of various lifestyle conditions as it displays a more concerted strategy in which the therapist explores the client's personal discouragements [17]. Therefore, motivational interviewing requires skills/training of the care provider and more time resources than the other approaches [2, 14]. It is also noteworthy, however, that sociocultural factors may influence motivational interviews. For instance, the acceptance of motivational interviewing as a therapeutic process may be undermined by someone from a culture that believes in medication for every therapy [14]. Hence, the clinician must explore all areas of the client's ambivalence for the motivation technique to be effective.

Similarly, in the area of nutritional control in the management of chronic health conditions like sarcopenia, the physician or dietetic prescribes a dietary plan. That plan is passed in the form of health advice or education; but unfortunately, without motivation, the patient may soon quit the plan. The relationship between nutrition and sarcopenia has been studied with success, leading to specific nutritional recommendations [1, 9, 17]. Motivational interviewing, when compared with usual care which is based on patient education and advice, is reported to be more effective in changing the physical appearance of the patient [9, 14]. The motivational technique helps the sarcopenic client to progress through the "stages of change" and maintain positive behaviour that would culminate in positive health outcomes [2, 17, 21].

Evidence abounds of the benefits of motivational interventions for lifestyle changes ameliorating sarcopenia prevention and treatment. Motivation alone does not prevent or treat chronic diseases, but it builds on the individual's power of willingness to apply tactics of behaviour change for the prevention of chronic disorders in primary care. Consequently, it is wise for a clinician in primary care setting to be acquainted with the tenet of motivational interviewing.

5. A guide to motivational interviewing (MI) in the prevention of sarcopenia

Although there is a scarcity of evidence on sarcopenia prevention among geriatrics using motivational techniques, there is evidence suggesting that improvements in diverse lifestyle changes take effect from motivational interviewing (MI). Evidence suggests that physical activity and dietary control increase with MI among the elderly population at risk of chronic disorders like sarcopenia, thereby improving their quality of life [17].

Occasionally, there could be hindrances to the success of motivational techniques. Addressing these obstacles is the merit of motivational interviewing. For example, workout schedules require the consideration of the physical safety of a geriatric with regard to capability, availability of any workout gadget, and the nature of the environment. Non-ambulant elderly can benefit from chair exercises which is a combination of cardio and strength which may also benefit those with orthopaedic problems like osteoarthritis and spondylosis. Motivational techniques for geriatrics with mental health conditions such as depression, anxiety, or cognitive impairment could be done together with a mental health therapist. An additional obstacle to workouts is fluctuating blood glucose levels. Inactive elderly with type 2 diabetes mellitus commencing workout plans (either aerobic or strength) will experience noninsulin-dependent uptake of blood glucose because of muscular contractions. Hence, meal timing and drug prescription may need to be adjusted by the physician and the dietitian in conjunction with a geriatric exercise plan to prevent hypoglycemia. For this, the American Diabetes Association recommends a small carbohydrate snack be carried along. Patient careers and/or family members should be involved in the exercise plan to ensure safety and effectiveness [17, 21].

MI is a clinically acceptable therapy for persons requiring health behaviour change. Its initial usefulness was in solving substance use disorders but its contemporary usefulness has shown positive effects in diverse health problems requiring behaviour modification, especially in chronic diseases. The MI model views motivation as the element that evokes readiness to change but not as a personality trait [21]. MI technique is based on the following elements [22]:

a. A set of principles called the "The Spirit of MI" by the originators, Miller and Rollnick

b. A set of skills to tackle MI are referred to as the "Tools" for MI

c. Steps in MI which are a set of walk-way that cause the real lifestyle modification

d. Effective communication skills which is a set of caregiver-patient engagement through a partnership that evokes client adherence, collaboration, and satisfaction with lifestyle changes.

e. Practical interviewing skills are a set of tactics and methods to enhance communication bonds and relax the client. These skills have a long-term benefit in therapeutic engagement and the potential to make the patient freer to disclose required information and be openhearted to discussions.

f. Psychosocial risk factors are the psychological and social circumstances that tend to constitute barriers to the patient's ability to embrace and sustain behavioural change. These factors can be assessed by the therapist through an established question line, followed by other further questions frequently for extra clarification.

g. Therapeutic alliance is about the clinician's understanding of a particular patient's perception, awareness, and knowledge of beliefs and coping practices about specific behavioural risk factors. A strong therapeutic alliance can have positive effects on treatment outcomes for patients [2, 3].

The following illustrative steps below can be followed hypothetically in a case of prevention of sarcopenia using the succeeding motivational interviewing elements in an ideal primary care setting:

The initial requirement is the "spirit" of MI by the therapist. The mnemonic "PACE" becomes handy in reminding the user of the four sets of qualities to be demonstrated: partnership, acceptance, compassion, and evocation. In "*partnership*", the interviewer and patient collaborate. The general belief is that the clients are their own best therapists while the actual therapist works to assist with opening a discussion on possible preventive strategies but instructing the sarcopenic. In order to partner effectively with the patient, the therapist must be in "*acceptance*" of the client's individuality, personality and beliefs. Although the therapist should not ignore any unhealthy lifestyle in the client, the therapist must be unconfrontational, non-judgmental, and uncondemning of the patient. Instead, no matter the client's illness experience, the therapist must express empathy. This expression of "*compassion*" from the clinician is one of the most valuable aspects of therapeutic counselling. Finally in the spirit of MI, the therapist dialogues on the need for changing behaviour. The therapist should "*evoke*" the client's comprehension on the reasons and elements, to modify their lifestyle. The therapist can prompt inquisitiveness, in order to explore the client's fears, ideas and expectations.

A further requirement for the effective use of MI is the set of five tools which the therapist requires to be skilful. They consist of: *Expressing empathy* by being concerned about the circumstances of the clients, understanding and accepting the patient's context. This facilitates the councillor-client relationship and encourages a robust discussion. During the MI, the clinician displays *Avoiding arguments* skills. The therapist must be ready to handle conflicts in order to create an enabling environment for discussion. Also, by *Supporting self-efficacy,* the clinician may support or help to refine the patient's choices for lifestyle change. As a result, the patients would develop confidence in their resolve to change. Additionally, skills in *Developing goals* entails the patient taking responsibility for a planned task. The interviewer does not apply coercion in task setting but assists the patients in developing positive thoughts and beliefs. When the therapist gives constructive suggestions to the client without coercion in order to refine the client's perceptions, the clinician is *Rolling with resistance*.

The real path treaded by the therapist delivering MI to cause the actual change process is called the steps, which is a set of successive patterns displayed by the therapist. The interviewer begins by *Establishing rapport* by an open communication that natures mutual trust to relate with the client. Next is the need for *Setting the agenda* of the mutual interaction, aiming at realistic preventive or therapeutic task of motivation to change without coercion on the client. *Assess readiness to change* is a necessary step to classify the client's motivation based on the trans-theoretical model of the stages of change. Knowledge of the client's level of motivation (pre-contemplation, contemplation, action, or maintenance) assists the clinician with how to *Re-adjust the focus* of MI by ensuring that by the therapeutic encounter the gets motivated and moves from a lower to a higher stage of change. The clinician must identify the lifestyle that requires change. By doing so, the clinician assists the client to *Identify uncertainty* which can be an obstacle to the client's motivation to change. The clinician then takes the responsibility to *Encourage self-motivation* in the patient by harbouring a positive mindset and clamouring for success.

Another element of motivational interviewing is *Effective communication*. This element assists the clinician in both patient assessment and motivational therapy because an effective communication strategy can engender a robust bonding between the therapist and the patient. By bridging any relationship gap, this element portends the potential of prompting patient disclosure of information as the consultation proceeds. An effective communication may be in the form of verbal or non-verbal communication. Non-verbal communication is based on gestures, hence it is also called body language and it is perceived to be a more potent and dependable means of communication. Both communication types are usually in agreement and the therapist should correctly reply to them at all times. This is because clients discuss more openly when they feel appropriately replied. The strategy of mimicking or matching the patients' gestures renders them more comfortable with their actions when it is done logically, respectfully, not disdainful or demeaning manner. The body language of a patient is a valid communication in all settings. On the other hand, verbal communication is the sum of all spoken exchanges between the patient and the therapist from the beginning to the end of the encounter. This communication type depends on the interviewing skills described by the OARS mnemonic. These skills can be improved upon with practice. In this method, through bonding with the clients, the clinician assists the patient to self-reflect and be open to discussion in the therapeutic process. The elements in this technique include these four: *open-ended questions* entail chaperoning the client into reflective thinking using open-ended questions which do not have preemptive answers. *Affirmation* is the process during which the interviewer validates the client's efforts and success thereby motivating the client to make an effort to accomplish more in the therapy process. In continuation, the therapist engages in *reflective listening* for further understanding of the discussion by giving a thought on the discourse with the client. The therapist then *summarises* the patient's point of view to ensure nothing said is missing. Since the patients are considered their own experts, the clinician is therefore never to presume a patient's thoughts or beliefs.

In Physiopedia [3], "Practical application of motivational interviewing", it is strongly suggested that the therapist needs to be in charge of the therapeutic interview. This can be achieved by signposting. Signposting is a verbal indicator of the direction taken as the therapist subjectively assesses the clients in order to help them move through different thoughts, stay focused, and be involved. For this, phrases and words are used to guide the patient through the consultation. Two main types of signposting are frequently used: (1) introductions/conclusions, and (2) outlining the main arguments or the direction of the argument in the discussion. Signposting skill is useful in keeping track of the planned agenda when the patient is going off topic. Also, clinical interviewers are expected to imbibe communication attributes like speaking slowly, and deliberately, asking brief questions, making one inquiry at a time, and using "words that heal". Medical jargon should be avoided during therapeutic discussions with patients, and the concerns of the patient should be well understood alongside the volume of information about their health they can afford to handle. Some common mistakes that should be avoided in verbal communication include, but are not limited to the following: *Bias:* occasionally, individuals are receptive to ideas while others are not. During inquiries, the therapists should try not to show their bias while interviewing. For instance, when a yes answer is being anticipated, a question with a bias towards no is asked. Just like during interviewing about home workout schedule, a question like: "did you enjoy your exercises?" is rather closed-ended and inclined towards the affirmative, while a question like: "I know you are a busy one, how were you able to achieve some workouts this week?", is open-ended and eliminates much bias. *Brevity:* This entails making inquiries using brief and direct queries to evade misperception and misconception. Open ended questions may be asked, but basically the patient is allowed to intensely communicate. *Spontaneous Information:* This is frequently required to grant the care provider the inkling about the client's behaviour thereby helping to clarify the background of the client's sarcopenia experience. *Keywords:* Occasionally the client's response contain specific message; hence, it is wise to explore the key point early as the patients communicate their context. As soon as the therapist elucidates the keyword, signposting

DOI: http://dx.doi.org/10.5772/intechopen.1005874

is used to maintain the interaction in line with the planned agenda. *Errors in Verbal Communication:* It is important for the therapist to correctly infer the client's opinions. In doing this, the therapist needs to intermittently confirm the clarity of what is understood in the patient's words. Consequently, the following three are key areas the therapist may need to clarify during the therapeutic communication: *Unclear statements:* This entails the therapist remembering to check whether the patient is on the same page as he or her by asking if the clients have any questions. *Misinterpreting:* Often, the therapist can be unfamiliar with the patient's language occasionally leading to misunderstanding the patient's communication. If the interview is not conducted in the patient's main language, there may be additional communication challenges. The therapist needs also to maintain a neutral and sensitive position not condemning the patient's views. *Assuming:* The care provider also, should not be haughty in the interaction. For example, if a patient complains that: "The pain never goes away", then that serves as a good opportunity to delve into the 24-hour pain inventory of related factors. This helps provide a clear picture to the therapist of possible true red flag or if emotions/other factors are affecting the description of their experience.

Whereas the traditional behavioural therapeutic approaches emphasise much on features like intensity, duration, pattern, and nature of the health condition, it is however a worthy adventure in the MI approach to inquire about the patient's beliefs related to their symptoms, as well as their perspectives about their illness experience—including the therapy, together with their fears and expectations with regards to recuperating. To this end, the motivational interviewer needs to bear in mind to assess the client's psychosocial risk factors, another important element of MI counselling. During the assessment, the acronym, ABCDEFW, becomes handy for recalling the questions used in identifying potential psychosocial risk factors. The acronym means: "Attitudes and Beliefs; Behaviours; Compensation Issues; Diagnosis and Treatment; Emotions; Family; and Work". The aforementioned features were described by Louis Gifford, 2014, suggesting that those psychosocial domains provide useful information about the patient behaviour and the illness behaviour characteristics that need to be understood for proper therapy to be given.

The following questions can help to guide the attending primary care physician, who needs to first reflect on possible answers, prior to asking the patient from the beginning of the MI session [3]:

- What information would be essential?
- Why would that information be necessary?
- How can it be phrased for proper understanding?
- How would this understanding affect the examination or treatment?
- What are possible outcomes?

By asking "Immediate Response Questions", the kind of inquiry that instigates the patient blurting out their concerns from their first answer, the physician then explores the patient's thoughts, idea, fears and expectations regarding their symptoms experience through a thorough questioning to translate the patient's actual worries into a therapeutic discussion. Below are some examples of helpful phrases and questions [3]:

- How does that compare with...?
- Is there any difference between...?
- How may I assist you with...?
- What is your idea about...going on...?
- What is your expectation of what should be done for...?
- Why do you think so about...?
- What do you think would help you feel better?
- How do you foresee your condition in the near future with regard to...?
- What did you find most helpful for your...?
- How do you feel about being dependent on others for assistance because of your condition?
- What makes you to have hope?
- What is your expectation?
- Assuming that in a snap all your symptoms suddenly change and you improved what things that you have given up on would you do again?
- How has your health condition affected your social network?
- Is the condition making you bitter about anything or person? Tell me about it.
- Can you share with me you feel by anyone talking about your condition that: "you are just making it up" or "it's in your head?"

Therapeutic alliance being another element of MI can have a strong positive effect on prognosis following behavioural therapy [3, 9, 11]. The therapist, being cognisant of the need for patients to deal with problems, perceive their problems in the right perspective, and despite their condition, navigate their activities of daily living, is prepared to effectively handle such patients [8, 12]. If the interaction *ab initio* is not effective, that divergent knowledge and beliefs may hamper with the therapeutic alliance [3]. Hence, it becomes necessary for therapists to appreciate the patient's context—they must be aware of patient-specific beliefs and associated risks. This will guide the therapists in educating the patients to understand the biomedical perspective of their condition—the therapeutic neuroscience education (TNE) approach [3].

The interaction tactics used during a therapeutic engagement should enhance patients' participation, and empower them to become engaged in both "problem-posing" and "problem-solving" endeavours [12]. Motivational interviewing (MI) communication strategies should enhance the sarcopenic patient's confidence, as well as their competence to make autonomous decisions [3]. It has been found that when clinicians with good communication skills engage with patients in MI, "patients are more satisfied with the care they receive, and the patients remember and demonstrate better knowledge; also, the therapist experiences more job satisfaction and less burnout" [3].

To sum up, a spirit harbouring tools, walking in guided steps, engaging effective communication skills in an everyday engagement to circumvent psychosocial barriers in order to conjure a therapeutic alliance of positive effects, is what MI is all about. Being a patient-centric, goal-directed, behavioural therapeutic approach, MI has the prospects of being a useful sarcopenia prevention and treatment tool in primary care settings. Some scenarios of MI usefulness in the primary care of sarcopenia, as have been discussed above, comprise the following postulations:

- Increasing physical activity: through MI, the primary care physician motivates geriatric patients to engage in regular exercise thereby promoting their muscle strength and function.

- Maintaining a healthy lifestyle: MI motivates the patient to live healthy by adopting and maintaining habits like healthy nutrition and stress management which generally support muscle health.

- Treatment programme retainership: geriatrics on prescribed workout and dietary regimens who receive MI, are more likely to adhere, thus enhancing the effectiveness of sarcopenia management.

- Behavioural change: MI enables the geriatric to initiate, progress and maintain long-term lifestyle practices that culminate in slower or halted progression of sarcopenia, giving rise to a valid prevention.

- Patient self-efficacy: through the therapeutic neuroscience education approach, MI empowers patients with life skills to self-manage and be in control of their symptom experience in sarcopenia care.

- Early intervention: by being a primary care tool, the MI therapeutic approach is initiated in the early stage of sarcopenia or its risks, potentially delaying sarcopenia progression or onset respectively.

While MI shows promise in sarcopenia primary care, further research is needed to fully explore its effectiveness in these contexts.

Author details

Katdel Istifanus Dafup
David Umahi Federal University Teaching Hospital, Uburu, Ohoazara,
Ebonyi State, Nigeria

*Address all correspondence to: katdeldafup@yahoo.com

References

[1] Kandayah T, Safian N, Azhar Shah S, Abdul Manaf MR. Challenges in the management of sarcopenia in the primary care setting: A scoping review. International Journal of Environmental Research and Public Health. 2023;**20**(6):5179. DOI: 10.3390/ijerph20065179

[2] Won CW. Management of sarcopenia in primary care settings. Korean Journal of Family Medicine. 2023;**44**(2):71

[3] Physiopedia. Practical Application of Motivational Interviewing [Internet]. 2023. Available from: https://www.physio-pedia.com/Practical_Application_of_Motivational_Interviewing [Accessed: January 24, 2024]

[4] Bruyère O, Reginster JY, Beaudart C. Lifestyle approaches to prevent and retard sarcopenia: A narrative review. Maturitas. 2022;**161**:44-48

[5] Rom Rom O, Kaisari S, Aizenbud D, Reznick AZ. Lifestyle and sarcopenia-etiology, prevention, and treatment. Rambam Maimonides Medical Journal. 2012;**3**(4):e0024. DOI: 10.5041/RMMJ.10091

[6] Feike Y, Zhijie L, Wei C. Advances in research on pharmacotherapy of sarcopenia. Aging Medicine (Milton). 2021;**4**(3):221-233. DOI: 10.1002/agm2.12168

[7] Castellano-Tejedor C. Non-pharmacological interventions for the management of chronic health conditions and non-communicable diseases. International Journal of Environmental Research and Public Health. 2022;**19**(14):8536

[8] Askin C, Baraki A, Feigenbaum J, Williams PN, Brigham SK, Watto MF. #186 Sarcopenia: Raising the Bar in Primary Care. The Curbsiders Internal Medicine Podcast. Available from: http://thecurbsiders.com/episode-list; 2019

[9] Alliance for Aging Research. Sarcopenia Research—Final Report [Internet]. 2022. Available from: https://www.agingresearch.org/wp-content/uploads/2023/03/AIM-Sarcopenia-Research-Final-Report.pdf [Accessed: January 24, 2024]

[10] Edwards HR, Jones H, Moseley J, Marshall T, El-Khamisy S, Aung MN, et al. Exercise interventions for the management of sarcopenia: Possibilities and challenges. Physical & Occupational Therapy in Geriatrics. 2 Oct 2023;**41**(4):654-677

[11] Yasuda T. Selected methods of resistance training for prevention and treatment of sarcopenia. Cells. 2022;**11**(9):1389. DOI: 10.3390/cells11091389

[12] Beaudart C, McCloskey E, Bruyère O, et al. Sarcopenia in daily practice: Assessment and management. BMC Geriatrics. 2016;**16**:170. DOI: 10.1186/s12877-016-0349-4

[13] Vaccaro JA, Gaillard T, Huffman FG, Vieira ER. Motivational strategies to prevent frailty in older adults with diabetes: A focused review. Journal of Aging Research. 2019;**2019**(1):3582679

[14] Taylor NF, O'Halloran PD, Watts JJ, Morris R, Peiris CL, Porter J, et al. Motivational interviewing with community-dwelling older adults after hip fracture (MIHip): Protocol for a randomised controlled trial. BMJ Open. 2021;**11**(6):e047970

[15] Pascual-Fernández J, Fernández-Montero A, Córdova-Martínez A,

Pastor D, Martínez-Rodríguez A, Roche E. Sarcopenia: Molecular pathways and potential targets for intervention. International Journal of Molecular Sciences. 2020;**21**(22):8844

[16] Cacciatore S, Massaro C, Landi F. Preventing osteoporosis, sarcopenia and obesity to care about quality of life. Annals of Geriatric Medicine and Research. 2023;**27**(1):87-90. DOI: 10.4235/agmr.22.0158 Epub 2023 Feb 27

[17] Sampaio RA, Sampaio PY, Uchida MC, Arai H. Management of dynapenia, sarcopenia, and frailty: The role of physical exercise. Journal of Aging Research. 2020;**2020**:8186769

[18] Maniar S, Bittner V. Lifestyle interventions for primary and secondary prevention of cardiovascular disease. In: PanVascular Medicine. Berlin, Germany: Springer Berlin Heidelberg; 2015. pp. 1695-1718

[19] Brinks J, Fowler A, Franklin BA, Dulai J. Lifestyle modification in secondary prevention: Beyond pharmacotherapy. American Journal of Lifestyle Medicine. 2016;**11**(2):137-152. DOI: 10.1177/1559827616651402

[20] Tokarek J, Kapuścik A, Kućmierz J, Kowalczyk E, Karbownik MS. Personality traits and health-related behaviors in medical students facing a stressful event. Frontiers in Public Health. 2023;**11**:1256883. DOI: 10.3389/fpubh.2023.1256883

[21] Donohue M. Benefits of Motivational Interviewing for Older Adults [Internet]. 2022. Available from: https://bluemoonseniorcounseling.com/benefits-of-motivational-interviewing-for-older-adults/ [Accessed: January 08, 2024]

[22] Miller WR, Rollnick S. Motivational Interviewing: Helping People Change. Guilford Press; 2012